AROMATHERAPY

A Complete Guide to the Healing Art

Alternative Medicine Series No. 1

AROMATHERAPY
A Complete Guide to the Healing Art

Kathi Keville and Mindy Green

Sri Satguru Publications
A Division of
Indian Books Centre
Delhi, India

Published by :
Sri Satguru Publications
A Division of :
Indian Books Centre
Indological and Oriental Publishers
40/5, Shakti Nagar,
Delhi-110007
(INDIA)
email:ibcindia@ibcindia.com
Website: http://www.ibcindia.com/

We would like to acknowledge the efforts of all those in the field of aromatherapy and herbal education who work to promote personal and planetary healing through the use of plant medicines.

Sincere thanks to all those who helped make this book possible: Evelyn Leigh, Ron Stringer, Julia Fischer and Mary Greer, for their editing suggestions; Marianne Griffeth, for her samples and technical information; Kurt Schnaubelt, for his contributions, generosity, and patience with endless questions; Bob Glendenning, for his artistic direction; John Maginnis, for the beautiful photographs; John Steele, for his inspiration and teachings; Galina Lisin, for her technical editing; Jean-Claude Lapraz, Daniel Penoel and Pierre Franchomme, for their contributions to aromatherapy research and education (many of their teachings are reflected in this book); Robert Tisserand, for technical information; and to our students, who are always an inspiration to both of us.

—Mindy Green and Kathi Keville

Special appreciation to Galina Lisin, who had endless suggestions for improving this work. Heartfelt love and gratitude to my grandmother Alice Solem, for her encouragement, support and faith in my abilities. I'd especially like to honor Rosemary Gladstar, for her inspiration and guidance in my lifelong work with plants.

—Mindy

My heartfelt appreciation to Ron Bertolucci for his support and assistance in making this book a reality, for his skill in blending fragrances, and for sharing with me his passion for aromatherapy.

-Kathi

Interior design by Victoria May
First Indian Edition : Delhi, 1999
ISBN 81-7030-602-7

Published by Sunil Gupta for Sri Satguru Publications a division of Indian Books Centre, 40/5, Shakti Nagar, Delhi-110 007, India and printed at Mudran Bharati,Delhi 110 009.

Contents

PART III: ALCHEMY

PART IV: CHARTS

PART V: APPENDICES

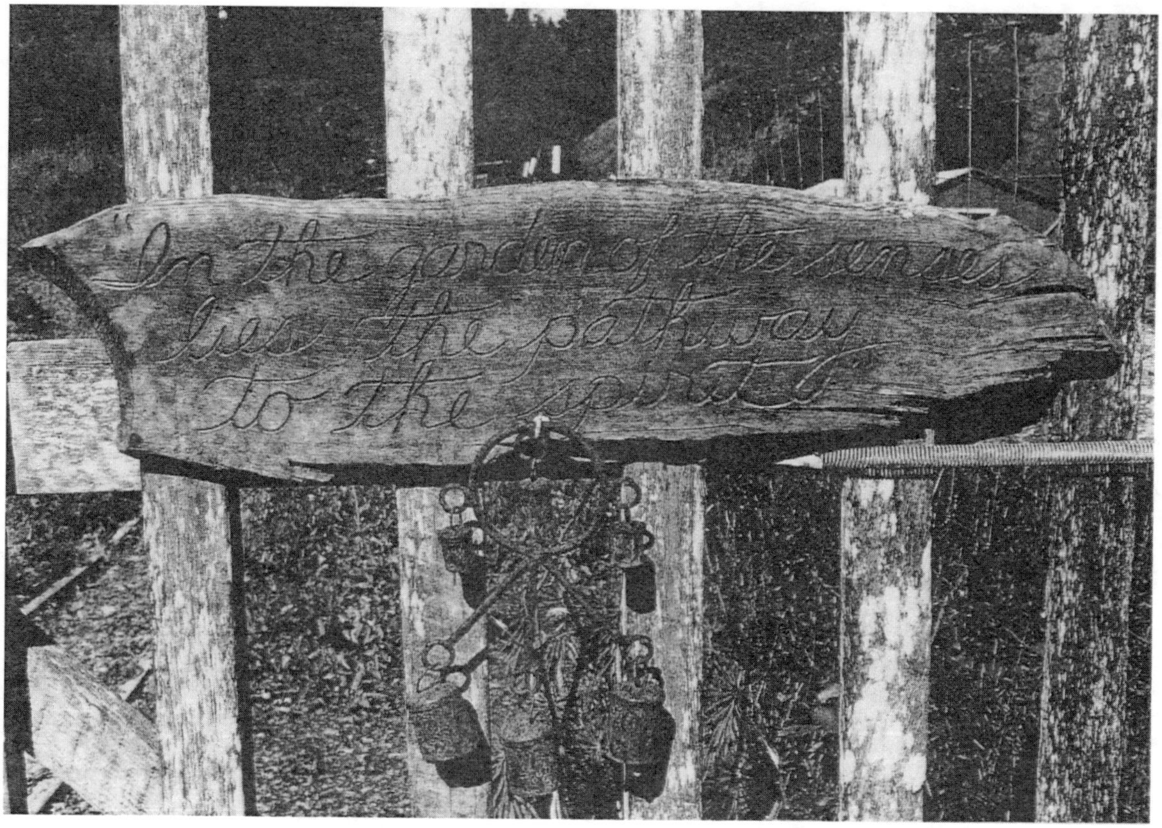
"In the garden of the senses
lies the pathway
to the spirit"

I'll never forget the first time I smelled the fruity fragrance of essential oil of carrot seed. I was instantly, dramatically and emotionally transported to my youth in the tropics. I saw myself as a child on a seesaw, surrounded by hundreds of mango trees. I could feel the humid tropical heat. I remembered the safe, carefree feeling of that moment. I felt again, and strongly, the love I had had for that place and for our housegirl, who served me that delicious fruit. All of this happened in an instant! In that brief moment, years of memories floated effortlessly back into consciousness—a clear example for me of the unconscious power of scent-association, memory and emotional programming.

—Mindy Green

As a child, I was drawn to the wonderful smells around me, and some of my most distinct memories are associated with those smells: my grandmother Irene's Chinese potpourri jar filled with rose petals, my grandmother Janna's cookie jar, the pine-scented woods where we went camping, the great variety of fragrant plants that abound in southern California, including the pungent sages of the desert. But my real exposure to olfactory delight began with my first herb garden. Every visitor who came by was dragged outside, usually without much protest, to sniff pineapple sage, coconut, geranium, lemon verbena and cinnamon basil. The potpourri of scents never failed to evoke plenty of smiles and dreamy, faraway gazes!

—Kathi Keville

Preface

The word "aromatherapy" conjures up images of people magically alleviating their depression or insecurities with wonderful scents. But aromatherapy is much more than that. Incorporating aromatherapy into your life enhances your overall health, beauty and psychological well-being. Aromatherapy can reduce stress, improve sleep and give you more energy. It can improve your complexion, treat an annoying skin itch and eliminate a stomachache.

Perhaps the best thing about aromatherapy is that is so easy and pleasurable to engage in. Few people will complain about receiving a prescription to bathe with scented oils or apply a fragrant body oil—two of the most popular aromatherapy techniques.

Essential oils give plants their characteristic odors, enabling us to take deep drafts of a fragrant rose bloom or drink in the perfume of lilacs and lavender. It is because essential oils are by their very nature aromatic that the therapy involving their use has been christened "aromatherapy."

There are two main ways to use fragrance in healing. One is through inhalation alone, which has its most significant impact on mood and emotion, but also produces physical reactions, such as lowered blood pressure. The other route is the physical application of essential oils to the body—by massage, for example, or by applying antiseptic oil to stop infection. Of course, any time you use an aromatherapy oil medicinally it can't help but do double duty: the fragrance is also inhaled.

Exactly how aromatherapy works is still unclear. Some researchers speculate that odors influence feelings because the nasal passage opens directly onto the part of the brain that controls emotion and memory. Others believe that fragrance compounds interact with receptor sites in the central nervous system. Psychic healers believe that fragrances work on subtle, still undiscovered energies in the body.

What we do know is that merely smelling a fragrance can influence us physically and emotionally by altering hormone production, brain chemistry, stress levels and general metabolism, as well as by affecting thoughts and emotions.

There are many good books on herbs and aromatherapy, but few (if any) address their joint application. Encouraged by our combined 45 years' experience studying and teaching the healing uses of plants, we decided to combine our efforts and write about aromatherapy from the herbalist's perspective. We hope that this book conveys our enthusiasm, love and appreciation of plants in all their variety, and that it inspires you to connect more deeply with the green world. May aromatherapy be as much of a healing journey for you as it has been for us!

It is an inspiration for us to see people get excited about the aromas and healing powers of plants. If you wish to become more familiar with plants, we recommend that you observe them in nature, grow them, taste them (cautiously), pick and dry them, and use them to make your own medicine. Most of all, give thanks for them.

PART I

Theory

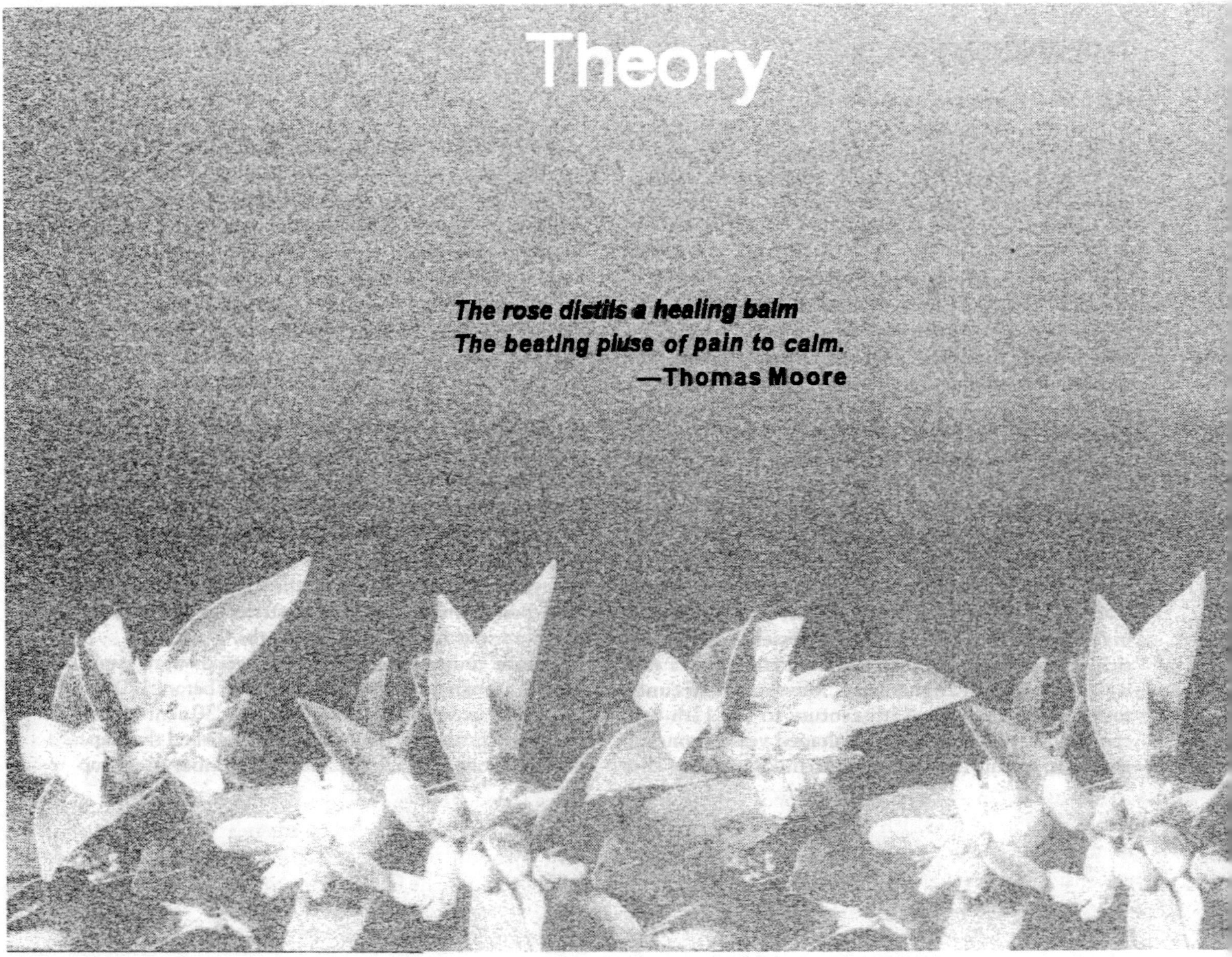

The rose distils a healing balm
The beating pluse of pain to calm.

—Thomas Moore

1

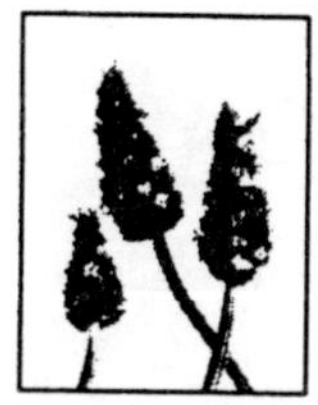

A History of Fragrance

THE ANCIENT WORLD

Much of the ancient history of fragrance is shrouded in mystery. Anthropologists speculate that primitive perfumery began with the burning of gums and resins for incense. Eventually, richly scented plants were incorporated into animal and vegetable oils to anoint the body for ceremony and pleasure. From 7000 to 4000 BC, the fatty oils of olive and sesame are thought to have been combined with fragrant plants to create the original Neolithic ointments. In 3000 BC, when the Egyptians were learning to write and make bricks, they were already importing large quantities of myrrh. The earliest items of commerce were most likely spices, gums and other fragrant plants, mostly reserved for religious purposes.

While on a modern archeological expedition in 1975 to the Indus Valley (which runs the length of modern Pakistan), Dr. Paolo Rovesti found an unusual terra-cotta apparatus, displayed along with terra-cotta perfume containers, in a Taxila museum. It looked like a primitive still, although the 3000 BC dating would place it 4,000 years earlier than most sources date the invention of distillation. Then a vessel of similar design, from around 2000 BC and unquestionably a still, was discovered in Afghanistan. Mesopotamian cuneiform tablets from the 13th century to the 12th century BC describe elaborate egg-shaped vessels containing coils; again, their function is unknown, but they are quite similar to Arab *itriz* used much later in the history of the region for distillation.

Even if essential oils were available at such an early date, most man-made fragrance was still in the form of incense and ointments. During the reign of the Egyptian pharaoh Khufu, builder of the Great Pyramid (c. 2700 BC), papyrus manuscripts recorded the use of fragrant herbs, choice oils, perfumes and temple incense, and told of healing salves made of fragrant resins. Throughout the African continent people coated their skin with fragrant oils to protect themselves from the hot, dry sun. This practice extended to the Mediterranean, where athletes were anointed with scented unguents before competing.

From this same era, the *Epic of Gilgamesh* tells of the legendary king of Ur in Mesopotamia (modem Iraq) burning *ntyw*, incense of cedarwood and myrrh to put the gods and goddesses into a pleasant mood. A tablet from neighboring Babylonia contains an import order for cedar, myrrh and cypress; another gives a recipe for scented ointments; a third suggests medicinal uses for cypress. Still farther east, the *Chinese Yellow Emperor Book of Internal Medicine*, written in 2697 BC, explains various uses of aromatic herbs.

Trade routes to obtain fragrant goods were established throughout the Middle East well before 1700 BC and would be well-traveled for the next 30 centuries—until the Portuguese discovered a way around the Cape of Good Hope. The Old Testament describes one group of early traders: "a company of Ishmaelites [Arabs] from Gilead, bearing spicery, balm and myrrh, going to carry it down to Egypt." Perhaps as early as 1500 BC, monsoon winds began carrying double-outrigger canoes along the "cinnamon route."

Egypt's penchant for producing unguents and incense was to become legendary. A figure of King Thothraes IV, carved into the base of the Sphinx at Giza, has been offering devotional incense and oil libations since 1425 BC, and there is little doubt that Egyptian aromas were potent: calcite pots filled with spices such as frankincense preserved in fat still gave off a faint odor when opened in King Tutankhamen's tomb 3,000 years later. As depicted on wall paintings, solid ointments of spikenard and other aromatics, called "bitcones," were placed on the heads of dancers and musicians, where they were allowed to gradually—and dramatically—melt down over hair and body.

The most famous Egyptian fragrance, *kyphi* (the name means "welcome to the gods"), was said to induce hypnotic states. The City of the Sun, Heliopolis, burned resins in the morning, myrrh at noon and *kyphi* at sunset to the sun god Ra. *Kyphi* had more than religious uses, however. It could lull one to sleep, alleviate anxieties, increase dreaming, eliminate sorrow, treat asthma and act as a general antidote for toxins. Several recipes are recorded, one of the oldest being a heady blend of calamus, henna, spikenard, frankincense, myrrh, cinnamon, cypress and terebinth (pistachio resin), among other ingredients. Cubes of incense were prepared by mixing ground gums and plants with honey, similar to a technique used by the Babylonians and later adapted by both Romans and Greeks.

The ancient Hebrews employed fragrance to consecrate their temples, altars, candles and priests. The book of Exodus (c. 1200 BC) provides the recipe for the holy anointing oil given to Moses for the initiation of priests: myrrh, cinnamon and calamus, mixed with olive oil. Although Moses decreed severe punishment for anyone who obtained holy oils and incense for secular use, not all aromatics were restricted to religious use. We learn in the book of Proverbs that "ointment and perfume rejoice the heart" (27:9), while in the Song of Solomon we read:

A bundle of myrrh is my beloved unto me;
He shall lie all night between my breasts
My beloved is unto me as a cluster of camphire [henna]
In the vineyards of En-gedi. (1:13-14)

By the late 5th century, Babylon was the principal market for the perfume trade. The Babylonians used cedar of Lebanon, cypress, pine, fir resin, myrtle, calamus and juniper extensively. When the Jews returned from captivity in Babylon, they brought back a heightened appreciation of fragrance, especially in the form of incense.

The ancient Greek world was also rich in fragrance. Just one Greek word, *arómata*, describes incense, perfume, spices and aromatic medicines. One such concoction, manufactured by a perfumer named Megallus, was the legendary *megaleion*, which contained burnt resin, cassia, cinnamon and myrrh, and was used in the treatment of wounds and inflammation. At Delphi, the oracle priestesses sat over smoldering fumes of bay leaves to inspire an intoxicating trance; holes in the floor allowed the smoke to "magically" surround them.

By the 7th century BC, Athens had developed into a mercantile center in which hundreds of perfumers set up shop. Trade was heavy in fragrant herbs such as marjoram, lily, thyme, sage, anise, rose and iris, infused into olive, almond, castor and linseed oils to make thick unguents. These were sold in small, elaborately decorated ceramic pots, similar to the smaller jars still sold in Athens today.

While Socrates heartily disapproved of perfume, worrying that it might blur distinctions between slaves (who smelled of sweat) and free men (who apparently did not), Alexander the Great—who, when he entered the tent of the defeated King Darius after the battle of Issos, contemptuously threw out the king's box of priceless ointments and perfumes—learned to love aromatics after a few years traveling in Asia. He sent deputies to Yemen and Oman to find the source of the Arabian incense with which he anointed his body and which burned constantly by his throne. To his Athenian classmate Theophrastus he sent plant cuttings obtained during his extensive travels, thus establishing a botanical garden in Athens. Theophrastus' treatise *On Odors* covered all the basics: blending perfumes, shelf life, using wine with aromatics, properties that carry scent, and the effect of odor on the mind and body.

As trade routes expanded, Africa, South Arabia and India began to supply spikenard, cymbopogons and ginger to Middle Eastern and Mediterranean civilization; Phoenician merchants traded in Chinese camphor and Indian cinnamon, pepper and sandalwood; Syrians brought fragrant goods to Arabia. True myrrh and frankincense from distant Yemen finally reached the Mediterranean by 300 BC, by way of Persian traders. Traffic on the trade routes continued to swell as demand increased for roses, sweet flag, orris root, narcissus, saffron, mastic, oak moss, cinnamon, cardamom, pepper, nutmeg, ginger, costus, spikenard, aloewood, grasses and gum resins.

By the 1st century AD, Rome was going through about 2,800 tons of imported frankincense and 550 tons of myrrh per year. Nero, Roman emperor in 54 AD, spent the equivalent of $100,000 to scent just one party he was giving. Carved ivory ceilings in his dining rooms were fitted with concealed pipes that sprayed down mists of fragrant waters on guests below, while panels slid aside to shower guests with fresh rose petals. (All this fragrant excess wasn't without its casualties; one unfortunate guest is said to have been asphyxiated by a dense cloud of those petals.) Both men and women literally bathed in perfume while attended by slaves called *cosmetae*. Three types of perfume were applied to the body: solid unguents, scented oil and perfumed powders, all purchased from the shops of *unguentarii*, who were regarded every bit as highly as doctors. The Romans even referred to their sweethearts as "my myrrh" and "my cinnamon," much as we use the gustatory endearments "honey" and "sweetie pie."

The Roman historian Pliny, author of the impressive 1st-century AD *Natural History*, mentions 32 remedies prepared from rose, 21 from lily, 17 from violet and 25 from pennyroyal. Famous Roman blends of the era included *susinon*, which served not only as a perfume but was a diuretic and women's anti-inflammatory tonic, and *amarakinon*, used to treat indigestion and hemorrhoids, and to encourage menstruation. A similar spikenard ointment was suggested for coughs and laryngitis.

Fragrance occurs, at least symbolically, throughout the New Testament records. The frankincense and myrrh brought to the Christ child were more valuable than the gift of gold (if indeed it was gold; some New Testament scholars speculate that the three wise men may have been carrying gold-colored, fragrant ambergris). One of the most famous gospel scenes involves Judas Iscariot complaining about Mary Magdalene's anointing of Christ's feet with costly spikenard. Even the Greek word for Christ, *Christos*, means "anointed," from the Greek *chriein*, to anoint.

Indeed, the 1st century AD was a time of accelerated development of aromatherapy's source sciences. Aromatics was one of five sections covered in Dioscorides' famous *Herbal*. The first written description of a still in the Western world is of one invented by Maria Prophetissima and described in *The Gold-Making of Cleopatra*, an Alexandrian text from around the first century. (Her design was used initially to distill essential oils, but also proved useful for alcoholic beverages.) Gnostic Christians from the 1st to the 4th century AD, whose beliefs were deeply rooted in Egyptian philosophy, held fragrance in high regard. Seeking release from the limitations of the material world, they embraced the symbology of essential oils, which represented the soul of the plant.

ORIENTALIA

Distillation of essential oils and use of aromatics also progressed in the Far East. Like the Christian Gnostics, Chinese Taoists believed that extraction of a plant's fragrance represented the liberation of its soul. Like the Greeks, the Chinese had just one word, *heang*, for perfume, incense and fragrance. Moreover, *heang* was classified into six basic types, according to the mood induced: tranquil, reclusive, luxurious, beautiful, refined or noble.

The Chinese upper classes made lavish use of fragrance during the T'ang dynasties, which began in the 7th century AD, and continued to do so until the end of the Ming dynasty in the 17th century. Their bodies, baths, clothing, homes and temples were all richly scented, as were ink, paper, sachets tucked into their garments, and cosmetics. The ribs of fans were carved from fragrant sandalwood. Huge, fragrant statues of the Buddha were carved from camphor wood. Spectators at dances and other ceremonies could expect to be pelted with perfumed sachets. China imported jasmine-scented sesame oil from India, Persian rosewater via the silk route and, eventually, Indonesian aromatics—cloves, gum benzoin, ginger, nutmeg and patchouli—through India.

Numerous texts related to aromatherapy were published in China. The *Hsian Pu* treatise by Hung Chu (1100 AD) describes incense-making. The 16th century saw publication of the famous Chinese Materia Medica *Pen Ts'ao*, which discusses almost 2,000 herbs, including a separate section on 20 essential oils. Jasmine was used as a general tonic; rose improved digestion, liver and blood; chamomile reduced headaches, dizziness and colds; ginger treated coughs and malaria.

It was the Japanese, however, who turned the use of incense into a fine art, even though incense didn't arrive in Japan until very late, around 500 AD. (The Japanese by then had perfected a distillation process.) By the 4th to 6th century, incense pastes of powdered herbs mixed with plum pulp, seaweed, charcoal and salt were pressed into cones, spirals or letters, then burned on beds of ashes. Special schools taught (and still teach) *kodo*, the art of perfumery. Students learned how to burn incense ceremonially and performed story dances for incense-burning rituals.

From the Nara through the Kamakura Periods (710-1333), small lacquer cases containing perfumes hung from a clasp on the kimono. (The container for today's Opium brand perfume was inspired by one of these.) An incense-stick clock changed its scent as time passed, but also dropped a brass ball in case no one was paying attention. A more sophisticated clock announced the time according to the chimney from which the fragrant smoke issued. Geisha girls calculated the cost of their services according to how many sticks of incense had been consumed.

THE MIDDLE AGES

The spread of Islam helped to expand appreciation and knowledge of fragrance. Mohammed himself, whose life spanned the 6th and 7th centuries, is said to have loved children, women and fragrance above all else. His favorite scent was probably camphire (henna), but it was the rose that came to permeate Moslem culture. Rose water purified the mosque, scented gloves, flavored sherbet and Turkish delight, and was sprinkled on guests from a flask called a *gulabdan*. Prayer beads made from gum arabic and rose petals released their scent when handled.

Following the translation in the 7th century of the Western classics into Arabic, Arab alchemists in search of the "quintessence" of plants found it represented in essential oils. The *Book of Perfume Chemistry and Distillation* by Yakub al-Kindi (803-870) describes many essential oils, including imported Chinese camphor. Gerber (Jabir ibn Hayyan) of Arabia, in his *Summa Perfectionis*, wrote several chapters on distillation. Credit for improving (and sometimes, erroneously, for discovering) distillation goes to Ibn-Sina, known in the West as Avicenna (980-1037), the Arab alchemist, astronomer, philosopher, mathematician, physician and poet who wrote the famous *Canon of Medicine*. Essential oils were used extensively in his practice, and one of his 100 books was devoted entirely to roses.

The 13th-century text by Arab physician Al-Samarqandi was also filled with aromatherapeutic lore, with a chapter on aromatic baths and another on aromatic salves and powders. Steams and incenses of marjoram, thyme, wormwood, chamomile, fennel, mint, hyssop and dill were suggested for sinus or ear congestion. Herbs were burned in a gourd, breathed as vapors, or sprinkled on hot stones or bricks. In India, the 12th-century text *Someshvara* described a daily bath ritual in which fragrant oils of jasmine, coriander, cardamom, basil, costus, pandanus, agarwood, pine, saffron, champac and clove-scented sesame oil were applied. Participants in Tantric ceremonies were also anointed with oils, the men with sandalwood, the women with a bouquet of jasmine on the hands, patchouli on the neck and cheeks, amber on the breasts, spikenard in the hair, musk on the abdomen, sandalwood on the thighs and saffron on the feet. In other rituals, women called *dainyals* held cloths over their heads to capture Tibetan cedar smoke, which would send them into prophetic chanting. Special finger rings held small compartments filled with musk or amber. Indian temple doors carved from sandalwood invited worshippers to enter (and conveniently deterred termites).

In Europe, a shining light of the Middle Ages was the Abbess of Bingen, Saint Hildegard (1098-1179), an herbalist whose four treatises on medicinal herbs included *Causae et Curae* ("Causes and Cures of Illness"), in which she spoke highly of fragrant herbs—especially of her favorite, lavender. (Some sources credit her with the invention of lavender water.) European nuns and monks closely guarded the formulas for "Carmelite water," which contained melissa, angelica and other herbs, and for *aqua mirabilis*, a "miracle water" used to improve memory and vision, and to reduce rheumatic pain, fever, melancholy and congestion.

From the 9th century to the 15th century, the Medical School of Salernum (Salerno) in Italy drew scholars from both the West and the East and crowned its graduates with bay-laurel wreaths. Here much Western knowledge, preserved and refined by the Moslems after the fall of Alexandria, was reestablished in the West. The school's *Regimen Sanitatis Salernitanum* was a kind of medical Bible for many centuries.

INFLUENCE OF THE SPICE TRADE

In the 13th and 14th centuries, Italy monopolized the Eastern trade established during the Crusades. The guilds—grocers, spicers, apothecaries, perfumers and glovers—controlled the import of enormous quantities of spices used to disinfect cities against the plague and other maladies. The purpose of Marco Polo's journey to China was to bypass Moslem middlemen and their 300-percent markup in price by convincing the Orient to trade directly with Genoa. When Christopher Columbus stumbled on the New World, he intended to make Spain a bigger player in the spice trade by beating out the competition. His route to the East was shorter. Tobacco, coca leaves, vanilla, potatoes and chilies of the Americas were of great interest to the rest of the world. Columbus kept looking for cloves and cinnamon but never did find these spices.

It was the good fortune of the Portuguese to finally establish a route around the tip of Africa, or "Cape of Storms" (later renamed "Cape of Good Hope"). In 1498, Vasco de Gama's sailors cheered, "*Christos e espiciarias!*" ("For Christ and spices!") as they neared India and her wealth of cloves, ginger, benzoin and pepper. (Jealous, Venice persuaded the Moslem traders to fight the Portuguese, who now controlled the spice trade. The Moslem traders were not successful.) The trade thus shifted from the Mediterranean to the Atlantic.

India—always prominent in the spice trade, although more as a pawn than a player—offered a rich variety of scents, including 17 types of jasmine alone. (The Moslem ruler Barbur, one of India's Mogul kings, declared, "One may prefer the fragrances of India to those of the flowers of the whole world.") The British, following the lead of the Dutch East India Company, finally attained a share of the action in the 18th century by taking control of India by exploiting the friction between the Moslems and Hindus. The British published an extensive set of volumes on medicinal and fragrant botanicals titled *The Wealth of India.*

THE AMERICAS

Columbus's assumptions were correct in one respect at least. The Americas indeed held fragrant treasures: balsam of Peru and Tolu, juniper, American cedar, sassafras, and tropical flowers like vanilla, heady with perfume. Like other indigenous peoples around the world, the Native Americans had a long history of burning incense and using scented ointments. Throughout the Americas, massage with fragrant oils was a common form of therapy.

The Aztecs were as extravagant with incense as the Egyptians, and they too manufactured ornate vessels in which to burn it. Injured Aztecs were massaged with scented salves in the sweat lodges, or *temazcalli.* The Incas made massage ointments of valerian and other herbs thickened with seaweed. In Central America, the Mayans steamed their patients one at a time in cramped clay structures.

Throughout the continent, North Americans "smudged" sick people with tight bundles of fragrant herbs or braided "sweet grass" (*Hierochloe odorata*), which smells like vanilla. Congestion, rheumatism, headaches, fainting and other ills were treated with smoke from burning plants, or with a strong herb infusion thrown over hot rocks to produce scented steam. The people of the Great Plains used echinacea as a smoke treatment for headaches; many tribes used pungent plants such as goldenrod, fleabane and pearly everlasting for therapeutic purposes.

SCENTS AND "SOPHISTICATION"

Even after losing control over the spice trade, Italy remained the European leader for cosmetics and perfumes. As Venice became more cosmopolitan, it began to produce scented pastes, gloves, stockings, shoes, shirts and even fragrant coins. Our word "pomander" comes from the French words *pomme d'ambre*, a scented ball made of ambergris, spices, wine and honey, carried in a perforated container carried on the belt or on a string around the neck. Dried medicinals were stored in beautiful porcelain pots, and botanical waters were kept in Venetian glass.

The Italian influence swept through France, helped along by Caterina de Medici's marriage to France's Prince Henri II. Making the journey with her were her alchemist (who probably also made her poisons too, but that's another story) and her perfumer, who set up shop in Paris. The towns of Montpellier and Grasse, already strongly influenced by neighboring Genoa, had long produced the perfumed gloves that were in high style among the elite. (The gloves were most often perfumed with neroli, or with animal scents such as ambergris and civet. Apparently this wasn't always appreciated. A 17th-century dramatist, Philip Massinger, complained: "Lady, I would descend to kiss thy hand/ but that 'tis gloved, and civet makes me sick.") These towns took the lead, as France's growing fragrance trade began to predominate over Italy's.

England was also influenced by the Italian love of scent. A pair of scented gloves so captured the attention of Queen Elizabeth I, she had a perfumed leather cape and shoes made to match. Sixteenth-century Elizabethans powdered their skin, hair and clothes with fragrant powders, and toned their skin with scented vinegars and fragrant waters. These waters like the Roman blends doubled as internal medicines.

The number of plants distilled expanded in the 16th century, and many books appeared on alchemy and the art of distillation. In 1732, when the Italian Giovanni Maria Farina took over his uncle's business in Cologne, he produced *aqua admirabilis*, a lively blend of neroli, bergamot, lavender and rosemary in rectified grape spirit. This was splashed on the skin, and also used for treating sore gums and indigestion. French soldiers stationed there dubbed it *eau de Cologne*, and Napoleon is said to have gone through several bottles a day—an endorsement that made it so popular that 39 competitors and a half century of law suits resulted. Other fashionable fragrances included rose, violet and patchouli, which were used on the imported Indian shawls made popular by Napoleon's famous consort, Josephine.

THE MODERN WORLD

In the 19th century, two important changes occurred in the Western world of fragrance. The 1867 Paris International Exhibition exhibited perfumes and soaps apart from the pharmacy section, thus establishing an independent commercial arena for "cosmetics." Even more significant was the production of the first synthetic fragrance, *coumarin* (which smells of new-mown hay), in 1868, followed 20 years later by musk, vanilla and violet. Eventually this list expanded to many hundreds, then thousands, of synthetic fragrances—the first perfumes unsuitable for medicinal use.

France became the leader in reestablishing the therapeutic uses of fragrance. The perfume industry had been divorced from medicinal remedies for 50 years, but slowly began to reclaim its medicinal heritage. The term "aromatherapy" was coined in 1928 by French chemist Rene-Maurice Gattefossé. His interest in using essential oils therapeutically was stimulated by a laboratory explosion in his family's perfumery business, in which his hand was severely burned. He plunged the injured hand into a container of lavender oil and was amazed at how quickly it healed.

By the 1960s, a few people, including the French doctor Jean Valnet and the Austrian-born biochemist Madame Marguerite Maury, were inspired by Gattefossé's work. As an army surgeon in World War II, Dr. Valnet used essential oils such as thyme, clove, lemon and chamomile on wounds and burns, and later found fragrances successful in treating psychiatric problems. But while Valnet helped inspire a modern aromatherapy movement when his book *Aromatherapie* was translated into English as *The Practice of Aromatherapy*, it was the appearance in 1977 of masseur Robert Tisserand's book *The Art of Aromatherapy*, strongly influenced by the work of Valnet and Gattefossé, that was successful in capturing American interest. At present, there are many books available on aromatherapy.

Most important, the efforts of pioneers like Valnet, Maury and Tisserand have turned aromatherapy into a disciplined healing art, rediscovering the uses of fragrance from ancient times and sparking a revival of aromatherapy that has swept throughout the world.

2

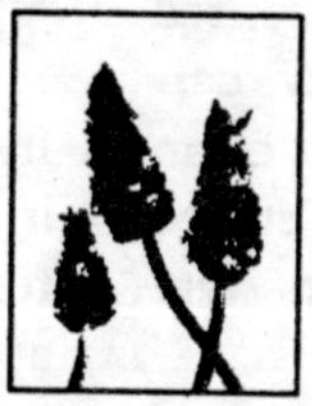

The Sense of Smell

Few things can move us so deeply or have so profound an impact on our psyches as the memories evoked by specific smells. A smell can take us back to childhood, conjure up a lost love or a sadness as real as the day we first experienced it. Smells invoke long-term memory and make the past present as none of the other senses can. The most direct of all our senses, smell has an immediate impact, uninfluenced by language and unimpaired by the passage of time.

Sensitivity to fragrance is to a large extent culturally determined, and there is no doubt that the culture in which we live influences our perceptions of which scents are "acceptable," "normal" or "pleasant." Primitive cultures have a much broader view of what is scent-acceptable. Members of one tribe in New Guinea say good-bye by putting a hand in each other's armpit, then rubbing themselves with the other's scent. Years ago, in the more highly developed culture of Japan, owing in part to the fact that Asians tend not to have as many apocrine glands at the base of their hair follicles as do people from the West, a strong body odor could disqualify men from military service.

Whatever your personal perceptions and preferences, there is no denying that the impact of odor is profound, if subtle. In her book, *Scent*, Annick LeGuerer wrote:

> Humans produce a characteristic odor in the air around them that reflects their diet and/or health, their age, their sex, occupation, race. It can be argued that because of the physiology of the olfactory apparatus, the most direct and profound impression we can have of another person is his (or her) smell. Indeed, smell bypasses the thalamus in the brain and penetrates directly to that organ's oldest part, the rhinencephalon, known to the Greeks as the "olfactory brain," where it produces, willy-nilly, pleasure or repugnance.

Smell is our most direct means of communion with nature. We smell with every breath we take, constantly monitoring the world around us, although we are not always conscious that we are doing so. (Just eight molecules of a substance can trigger an electrical impulse in a nerve ending, whereas roughly 40 nerve endings must be stimulated before we become conscious of any smell.) In the words of anthropologist Laurens Van Der Post, "Scent . . . is not only biologically the oldest but also the most evocative of all our senses. It goes deeper than conscious thought or organized memory and has a will of its own which human imagination is compelled to obey."

To fully understand aromatherapy and the effects of essential oils, we must arrive at a basic understanding of two physiological processes: how the olfactory apparatus works, and how essential oils are absorbed into the body.

HOW THE BRAIN PROCESSES ODOR

Odors are the effect of volatile molecules that float through the air, rushing through our nostrils as we inhale. There are three stages in the process of smelling. Fragrance begins with the *reception* of odor molecules, which, as they are inhaled, bind to the olfactory epithelium (receptor cells that contain, in all, some 20 million nerve endings). Odor *transmission* occurs when a message is fired to the right and left olfactory bulbs, located above and behind the nose at the base of the brain, each about the size and shape of a small lima bean. At this point a variety of cells and neurons interpret, amplify and transmit the message to the limbic system.

Perception takes place when the message is received by the hypothalamus. Acting as a relay station, the hypothalamus sends information to other parts of the brain, such as the pituitary gland, which sends chemical messengers into a) the bloodstream, b) the olfactory cortex, which helps distinguish odors, c) the thalamus, which helps connect odor messages with higher thought functions, and d) the neocortex, which finely analyzes odor messages, relating them to the other senses, as well as to the higher brain functions that stimulate conscious thought. All this happens in less than a second.

Recently Columbia University researchers isolated, for the first time in medical history, what they believe to be odor receptors. This large family of genes—perhaps numbering as many as 1,000—is much more complex than the three types of receptors the eye uses to distinguish a few thousand colors. The average adult can process about 10,000 different odors in an area of the brain about one inch square.

The sense of smell is crucial to the sense of taste. Where the tongue tastes only sweet, sour, salt and bitter, all other sensations perceived as taste are in fact odors. University of Texas taste physiologist Dr. James C. Boudreau believes that there may be more than 20 distinct human taste sensations, including bitter, two types of sweet, insipid, metallic, pungent, burning, warm and cool (as in menthol), astringent-dry and astringent-tangy.

Smell is the only sense with receptor nerve endings in direct contact with the outside world, providing a direct channel, as it were, to the brain. The "blood-brain barrier" is a lipid-rich (i.e., oil-rich) membrane that sheathes and protects the brain. Oxygen and some nutrients can pass through this membrane, but large molecules, such as those of most therapeutic drugs, cannot. Because the olfactory nerves evolved before the brain, they are not protected by this sheath.

The idea that something as noninvasive as natural odors can directly affect the mind is quite exciting. Medical researchers hope someday to be able to use this pathway to access specific areas of the brain with fragrance in order to treat various disorders, including Alzheimer's disease. For now, studies suggest that essential oils directly affect the central nervous system, modifying the brain's reactions.

The brain's response to a change in odor may be influenced by our thought patterns. Certain brain waves, called "contingent negative variation," or CNV, are very sensitive to emotional changes and are activated by particular fragrances. According to Robert Tisserand, different odors stimulate different brain centers to release neurochemicals (also called neurotransmitters) that affect us in a number of ways.

For example, "euphoric" odors such as clary sage and grapefruit stimulate the thalamus to secrete neurochemicals called enkephalins, natural pain killers that also produce a general feeling of well-being. Odors that stimulate the endorphin-secreting pituitary gland include the aphrodisiac scents jasmine and ylang-ylang. The pituitary also releases chemical messengers into the bloodstream to regulate other glands, such as the thyroid and the adrenals. Sedative odors such as marjoram stimulate the area of the brain called the "Raphe nucleus," triggering the secretion of the neurochemical serotonin, which helps us sleep.

ESSENTIAL OIL ABSORPTION THROUGH THE SKIN

As with absorption into the brain and central nervous system, the absorption of essential oils through the skin is quick and easy due to their lipid-solubility, to their extremely small molecular size and to the natural oiliness of the skin itself. Essential oils enter the bloodstream through small capillaries. They affect the nervous and lymphatic systems when they come in contact with nerve and lymphatic vessels in the dermal layer of the skin.

Studies show that after a full body massage with a 2-percent dilution of lavender essential oil in vegetable oil, detectable amounts of linalol and linalyl acetate, the main chemical constituents of lavender, are found in the blood. Concentrations were highest after 20 minutes and diminished to undetectable levels within 90 minutes. The study concluded that not only are essential oils lipophilic (oil soluble) by nature, but that massage with a fatty oil accelerates absorption of essential oils by the skin. You can experiment with this theory at home: garlic rubbed on the feet can later be smelled on the breath.

FRAGRANCE AND HEALTH

During the Black Plague in 17th-century Europe, stench was linked, quite naturally, to disease, decay and death. (In France, the term *peste* described both the disease and the odor associated with it.) People sniffed pomander balls and boxes containing cedarwood, and used hollow-topped walking sticks containing aromatic substances thought to ward off the plague. Nosegays were used for the same purpose; they were so popular that a London Bill of Mortality for 1635 gave precise instructions for their preparation. (The recipe included vinegar, rice, wormwood and rosewater.) "Strewing herbs" were spread upon the floor, their fragrance rising when crushed underfoot.

Many perfumers—and glove-makers, who perfumed their products—escaped the plague. We now know that their secret was the antibacterial properties of the essential oils they were exposed to in their daily work. It is said that Bucklersbury, England, was spared from plague because it was the center of the lavender trade, and even today the French city of Grasse, where so much perfume is produced, is known for having very low rates of respiratory illness.

Still, negative symptoms traceable to synthetic colognes and perfumes are increasing. These range from sinus pain to anaphylactic shock and seizures. The problem is a result of the increased strength of fragrances today, coupled with a rise in the use of synthetic chemicals. The U.S. Food and Drug Administration estimates that 4,000 different chemicals are currently used in fragrances, with a rise in the use of single perfume often containing several hundred chemicals. The FDA is particularly concerned about synthetic musk-like fragrances that have been associated with damage to the central and peripheral nervous systems.

The sense of smell has had a time-honored role in the diagnosis of disease. Typhoid fever is said to smell like freshly baked bread, diabetes like sugar, the plague like apples, yellow fever like a butcher shop, nephritis like ammonia. Chemist John N. Labows has a computer catalog of odor profiles to help identify infections. The Connecticut Chemosensory Clinical Research Center specializes in such diagnoses. In addition to exploring ways in which the sense of smell relates to aging, smoking, diabetes and other diseases, researchers there are also investigating how fragrance can be used to reduce the side effects of chemotherapy, kidney dialysis and radiation therapy.

Finally, there is new evidence that we may exercise direct control over health and disease through the hypothalamus. The way the immune system and the central nervous system operate is only vaguely understood, but researchers know that they do communicate with one another. Specific odors provide a pathway through the central nervous system that activates the immune system's protector cells. Current research suggests that it may be possible to teach the body to activate its own immune response by sniffing specific odors, although exactly which odors is not yet clear.

OLFACTORY DEPRIVATION

It is estimated that two million Americans have anosmia, the inability to smell or taste, a condition traceable to a number of factors. At the University of Pennsylvania Smell and Taste Center, 638 people were tested for their smell acuity. Not surprisingly, those who smoked had an olfactory deficit that corresponded to how much they smoked. Exposure to toxic chemicals can likewise cause a loss of taste and smell. In some instances a deficiency of the mineral zinc has been implicated in smell disorders, as well as in as some cases of infertility. Hormones, radiation, diet, drugs and the natural process of aging may also damage the sense of smell, as can antidepressants and anti-anxiety drugs, viral infection, head injury and menopause.

It is possible to increase your ability to smell by "scent exercising." Johns Hopkins researcher Robert Anholt found that most people have the potential to detect subtle differences in smell, but that it takes practice. Test subjects exposed themselves to as many natural odors as possible, thereby training their noses to recognize more scents. Supplements of the mineral zinc may prove helpful when the sense of smell is deficient.

ODOR AND EROS

In her book *A Natural History of the Senses*, Diane Ackerman wrote, "Because females have often been responsible for initiating mating, smell has been their weapon . . . " Perfumes reveal to the unconscious mind an aspect of sex appeal often hidden from consciousness. A kiss—the word means "smell" in many languages—is a prolonged sniffing of the loved one, an expression of the desire to linger where the beloved's scent glows.

Each of us has a unique personal odor, as individual as our fingerprints and influenced by diet, gender, heredity, health, medication, occupation, emotional state and mood. Personal odor communicates something about who we are and—instinctively and unconsciously, for better or for worse—is one of our criteria for choosing our friends and lovers. According to Dr. Susan Shiffman, "People who don't like each other's smell don't make it as a couple." North American culture, however, may be too acutely aware of body odor. Given our constant attention to removing odor with deodorants and replacing it with synthetic scents, researchers speculate that we may have lost our innate ability to respond to natural sexual attractants.

The odoriferous substances manufactured by the apocrine glands—found in the axillae (armpits), face, nipples, anal and genital regions, and to a lesser extent in the ears, eyelids and scalp—are called pheromones, from the Greek words *pherein* (to carry) and *hormon* (to excite). They become active at puberty, after which they play an interesting role in sexual behavior, puberty, menstruation and menopause. (Before puberty, perspiration has no odor, which makes perfect biological sense: there is no need to signal or attract the opposite sex before we are able to reproduce.)

There have been many interesting studies on how the sense of smell affects women. One study, for example, showed that girls who had been separated from boys during adolescence (in a boarding school situation) generally started menstruating later than girls in a coeducational environment. This suggests that contact with boys' pheromones triggers a hormonal response that signals girls to become fertile. Studies also show that women produce a pheromone that causes their menstrual cycle to synchronize with that of nearby women after three or four months. Women's sensitivity to odor peaks at ovulation, when olfactory receptivity increases a thousandfold. Conversely, women's sense of smell is least keen at menstruation.

The male underarm scent can also regulate women's cycles, although merely being in prolonged, close proximity is not enough to trigger this effect; there must be intimate physical contact. Other studies show that women who have sex with a male partner at least once a week have more regular menstrual cycles, are more likely to have cycles of normal length, have fewer infertility problems, and experience a milder menopause than women who are celibate or who have sex in a "feast or famine" pattern. Scientists are trying to isolate the chemicals responsible for these phenomena in order to produce nasal sprays for scent-based birth control and cycle regulation. Following menopause or hysterectomy, women lose their ability to detect musk odors, which are very close to human testosterone and can normally be detected in amounts as little as 0.000000000000032 ounces. (Twenty-five percent of people with smell disorders lose interest in sex; as part of their sex therapy, Masters and Johnson have helped couples learn to enjoy touching each other through the use of scented lotion.) The ability to detect musk odors is restored following hormone therapy. Fertile women who were exposed to a musk odor have shorter menstrual cycles, ovulate more often and conceive more easily.

Research offers little information on how scent affects men sexually. We found one reference to a scientist who lived in isolation for long periods on an island. By taking the dry weight of the hairs trapped by his electric razor every day, he discovered that his beard grew faster each time he returned to the mainland and associated with females. Although sex pheromones are produced by both men and women, the male sex pheromones seem to function mainly as aphrodisiacs for the female, whereas the female pheromones serve chiefly to announce her readiness.

Napoleon was keenly aware of how scent affects sexuality. It is reported that he once sent a message to Josephine that read, "Home in three days. Don't wash." Goethe carried around the unwashed bodice of his lover so as to never be without her fragrance. In Elizabethan times, lovers exchanged peeled "love apples," which were kept in the armpit until saturated with sweat, then presented to the lover so he or she could inhale the fragrance when they were apart. A similar custom was observed in parts of the Austrian Tyrol, where it was fashionable for a young man to dance with a handkerchief in his armpit and later wave it under the nose of the girl he admired to excite her sexually.

Studies show that females have, in general, a keener sense of smell than males, even as infants. Research by Hilary Schmidt of the Monell Chemical Senses Center in Philadelphia, while suggesting that the same odor preferences occur in both children and adults, also noted definite gender differences, with baby girls preferring scented rattles more often than baby boys. Another study showed that women could guess the sex of a person more accurately than men just by sniffing a shirt worn for 24 hours. Researchers also found that when women were given the male hormone testosterone, their ability to smell declined. In still another test, when puffs of fragrance were monitored by subjects, men performed better at simple mental tasks in unscented rooms while women did best in scented rooms. One group of male interviewers rated scented female applicants as less intelligent, albeit more attractive; when interviewed by women, fragrance-wearing female applicants were judged friendlier and more intelligent than those who wore no scent.

In 1974 Dr. Lewis Thomas—who advanced the theory that mate selection can be traced to individual odorprints generated by a sequence of genes—suggested that a cluster of animal genes known as the "major histocompatibilty complex" (MHC), which generates antibodies for protection, might be the key to the olfactory code. Immunologist Ted Boyse later proved the link between the sense of smell and the immune system by performing an experiment that demonstrated how MHC is influenced by smell. Working with strains of inbred mice, he was able to show that mice sniffed out genetically different mice with whom to mate, thus keeping the gene pool more diverse and establishing a more adaptable immune system. Mice even showed a preference to mate with those whose genetic makeup differed by only a single gene. A high variability in MHC is now thought to be essential for disease resistance.

3

Scent and Psyche

Manipulating fragrance to affect the emotions is nothing new. Ancient Egyptians and Greeks, followed later by Europeans, found that marjoram, cypress and hyssop were useful for comforting grief and sadness, "strengthening" the brain so the bereft individual could get on with his or her life. Sixteenth-century herbalist John Gerard recommended marjoram's fragrance "for those given to much sighing."

Today, realtors know that the aroma of a few freshly baked brownies, strategically placed and the fragrance from a few drops of essential oil on light bulbs improve the chances of selling a house. Used-car salesmen magically rejuvenate run-down autos with "new car" fragrance available in a can. Watch anyone buying body-care products. How do they make their final decision? They give the product a sniff, of course.

Fragrance is already being used experimentally in a few large U.S. department stores to see whether it will encourage people to spend. The director of the Smell and Taste Treatment and Research Foundation in Chicago, Dr. Alan R. Hirsch, says, "It is probable that by the year 2000 managers will use perfumes in department stores the world over . . . Odorants are potentially more efficacious than any other modality in increasing saleability."

Hirsch is busy comparing how different odors change consumers' reactions as they watch commercials for Oldsmobile cars or Nike running shoes. In another project, he piped appealing odors into the Las Vegas Hilton to see whether it would affect gamblers. Affect them it certainly did: people stayed longer, they spent more money, and revenues increased by 45 percent.

While aromatherapy research has tended to focus on marketing, it is also impacting medical science. (In this arena, it is usually identified by the slightly more scientific-sounding name "aromachology.") The 1990 International Conference on Essential Oils and Aroma Chemicals in Malaysia generated approximately 50 papers on the actions of essential oils. At the 1991 conference of the prestigious American Association for the Advancement of Science, the largest U.S. science organization, papers by aromachology researchers from major U.S. universities were delivered.

People tend to prefer familiar fragrances—that is, unless past negative associations get in the way. Researchers have demonstrated that odors with negative associations evoke negative emotions. When students at Warwick University in England were told they had performed poorly on a simple test they had taken while smelling a certain odor, they became depressed the next time they smelled that odor. Those who had been told they were successful had the opposite reaction: their self-confidence was boosted.

Most of the funding for scientific research into aromatherapy in the United States comes from the International Fragrance and Flavor (IFF) organization, a coalition of companies in the fragrance industry. This organization funded grants for clinical research which resulted in seven psychologists studying how the sense of smell functions, and how it affects mind and body. Researchers are particularly interested in discovering aromatic relaxants, stimulants, antidepressants and pain-relievers. Since these categories—"uppers" and "downers"—represent some of the most frequently prescribed drugs, the pharmaceutical industry may be in for a sea change.

Thanks to IFF funding, Dr. Craig Warren was able to test more than 2,000 subjects over a 20-year period to better understand how smell can relieve pain, touch off deep-seated memories, and affect personality and behavior. He is particularly interested in mood-elevating odors that prevent insomnia. Also sponsored by the IFF, Dr. Gary Schwartz of the University of Arizona believes that fragrances may provide valuable complementary treatment for a host of problems related to the emotions, such as fatigue, migraine headaches, food cravings, depression, anxiety, schizophrenia and irregular heartbeat.

Because the fragrance field is virtually married to the cosmetics industry, it should come as no surprise that modern aromatherapy was born of the quest for new and improved beauty products. A "Sleep for Beauty Kit" designed by the IFF in 1984 comes with a fragrant pillow and vials of 30 scents, such as neroli and valerian. The IFF's Henry D. Walter foresees more and more companies marketing perfumes designed to ease stress. Marina Munteanu, the IFF's fragrance-technology vice-president, projects that one day it will be commonplace for people to choose everyday scented items, such as shampoo, according to their emotional needs. Redken, a large cosmetics company, has already taken this marketing hint to heart and introduced its Shinsen hair line to "relieve stress and promote peace of mind" with rose, honeysuckle, tuberose and musk, or to "lift the spirits" with orange, tangerine and peach.

The first major cosmetics company to produce an aromatherapy line designed to influence the emotions was Avon with its "Tranquil Moments" bath products. Scientists at the Japanese fragrance firm Takasago, on the Avon payroll, measured brain-wave patterns and found that jasmine is stimulating, lavender relaxing—the same qualities attributed to these scents through centuries of folklore. (Takasago is currently investigating aromatherapy to relieve nausea, dizziness and other physical ailments.) Following Avon's lead, the Estée Lauder beauty company formed Origins, an aromatherapy body-care line sold in exclusive department stores. Their "Green Principles" products emphasize botanicals and carry names such as Sleep Time, Stress Buffer, Muscle Easing, Energy Boost and Peace of Mind.

The world's third largest cosmetics company, after Avon and Revlon, is a Japanese company called Shiseido whose name means "harmony among the natural forces that govern the world." Shiseido believes that beautiful skin begins with balanced *chi*, or life energy, and has put together an acupressure and aromatherapy facial with effects that are more than skin deep. Researchers found that the brain waves of subjects receiving aromatherapy facials duplicate those achieved during meditation or deep relaxation. Thus, in addition to improving the complexion and reducing acne, the facial stabilizes blood pressure, moderating both high and low readings.

Meanwhile, Charles of the Ritz has produced a fragrance to keep car and truck drivers alert. There is talk of extending this concept to air-traffic controllers and others who must stay alert while performing monotonous tasks. Train conductors in Japan and Russia already keep alert with an "odorphone" that spews out hot whiffs of rose and other floral scents—pine or cedar, even seaweed and mushroom. At least one New Zealand airline provides business and first-class passengers with a kit of floral-scented bath oils (from 50 different flowers) for use before and after flying to combat jet lag. (Princess Diana and Queen Elizabeth of England are reported to use these regularly in their jaunts around the world.)

Dr. Susan Schiffman, professor of medical psychology at North Carolina's Duke University, had certain food scents sprayed into New York City subway cars in order to observe the effect on passengers. After comparing the number of pushes, shoves and nasty comments in scented versus unscented cars, she concluded that fragrances can reduce such aggressive behavior by as much as 40 percent.

Aromatherapy products have found their way into a number of homes. A study of living-room environments sponsored by the fragrance company PPF/Norda indicated that participants react more favorably to furniture and decor when a room is fragranced. Robert

Baron, chairman of the Rensselaer Polytechnic Institute in Troy, New York, found that people perform a variety of tasks more accurately and efficiently in scented as opposed to unscented rooms. Clerical workers in one study set higher performance goals for themselves in scented offices.

The Japanese in particular have embraced aromatherapy and become leaders in innovative aroma applications. A futon-dryer that leaves the bedding smelling like flowers encourages sleep. After a good night's sleep, one may require the assistance of the Hattori Seiko alarm clock, which puffs pine and eucalyptus scent to gently rouse you just seconds before the sound alarm goes off). Japanese firms have also developed clothes impregnated with aroma beads, such as the lavender-and-rose scented pantyhose currently being sold on the European market.

Even house paint has entered the aromatherapy arena. City Surplus and Paint in Denver, Colorado, offers paints in more than a dozen mood-altering scents, including jasmine, pine and eucalyptus.

Aromatherapy has long had a role in the entertainment field. An "odor organ" in the early 20th century emitted different scents according to which keys were hit. The annual 1993 Comdex computer convention in Las Vegas displayed every kind of new computerized device, including a fragrance dispenser computer programmed to match the music's beat (and mood) as thousands of convention-goers danced. In London, a 1993 production of Prokofiev's *The Love of Three Oranges* added fragrance to the performance. The audience was cued when time came for them to release each of six odors on scratch-and-sniff cards. Hollywood had a similar idea in the early 1960s, when the first Smell-o-Vision movie houses, outfitted in New York City and elsewhere for the premiere of Michael Todd Jr.'s thriller *A Scent of Mystery*, ran pipes along the backs of theater seats that puffed out different scents as the plot progressed. (Unfortunately, they never got the timing right: the smell of perfume was apt to arrive long before the heroine, destroying suspense, and the premature smell of horses ruined at least one love scene.) Later, director John Waters would reinvent the scratch-and-sniff gimmick for his 1981 comedy *Polyester*.

FURTHER THERAPEUTIC APPLICATIONS

A 1992 issue of the *British Journal of Occupational Therapy* describes the potential of aromatherapy to "promote health and well-being" in hospital patients through massage, inhalation, baths, compresses, creams and lotions. According to the journal's extensive list of potential uses, aromatherapy can diminish stress, sedate, relieve depression, invigorate, promote activity and alertness, stimulate sensory awareness, facilitate interaction and communication, treat certain medical problems and provide pain relief. For years, anesthetists in many hospitals have used a strawberry fragrance on ether masks to calm children before surgery. In New York City, Memorial Sloan-Kettering Cancer Center is using vanilla scent to relax patients undergoing magnetic resonance imaging (MRI) scanning.

In England, similar aromatic methods are proving successful when used in conjunction with orthodox treatments to help patients cope with the emotional problems that may accompany serious illness. Aromatherapy is also used to diminish the side effects of drug therapies. Wirral Holistic Care Services, for example, currently uses aromatherapy to help cancer patients tolerate the side effects of chemotherapy (*Nursing Standard Journal*, 1991).

IFF studies have found that orange and other citrus scents reduce stress and depression. As aromatherapists, we have observed that some citrus scents are more effective than others, depending on the diagnosis. For example, true clinical depression responds better to the more refined scent of orange blossom, also known as neroli, than it does to orange peel. Lemon's "clean" fragrance helps maintain emotional balance. Bergamot helps overcome compulsive behavior, including eating disorders. Tangerine and grapefruit appeal to children subject to depression and mood swings, and assist adults doing "inner child" therapy.

ANXIETY AND STRESS

In his 17th-century *Herbal*, Nicholas Culpeper noted that chamomile "comforts both the head and brain."

We have found it particularly useful for treating children who are anxious or hyperactive, as well as stressed-out adults.

IFF-sponsored psychologist Dr. Gary Schwartz is studying how the sense of smell affects the area of the brain that regulates fear and anxiety. To achieve an initial increase in anxiety levels, the 48 people who participated in one experiment were asked provocative questions such as "What kind of person makes you angry?" As expected, the subjects tensed up—that is, until they sniffed an apple, whereupon their breathing became slower and their muscles relaxed. They felt happier, less anxious. Their systolic blood pressure rates fell a point, while diastolic rates went down three to five points. Adding a little spice—clove and cinnamon—to the apple heightened these effects.

When Dr. Paolo Rovesti, director in 1973 of the Instituto di Derivati Vegetali in Milan, used essential oils to treat depressed and anxious patients, he had success with fragrances considered "herbal" or "green," such as lavender, marjoram, violet leaf, rose, cypress and opopanax. Lavender turns out to be particularly effective in lowering anxiety and stress in patients following heart surgery. Aromatherapists use these same fragrances with people who are dealing with loneliness or rejection, or with anyone undergoing a major life transition.

IFF researchers have studied, and patented, two essential-oil blends to diminish anxiety and stress in the workplace. One is a combination of neroli, valerian and nutmeg; the other is from compounds found in essential oils: myristicin from nutmeg, elemicin and isoelemicin from elemi. Both blends, designed to be rubbed into the skin or inhaled, reduce stress and blood pressure. Individuals say they experience much less fear, tension and anxiety after sniffing them. Clinical studies have also found that smelling peaches reduces panic attacks, epilepsy and narcolepsy.

Dr. J. J. King, a psychiatrist who practices in Worcestershire, England, found that fragrance can break the feedback loop created during stress. When anxiety develops, heart and breathing rates increase, affecting brain chemistry, which in turn stimulates more anxiety. If this loop can be stopped by physical or psychological means, relaxation ensues. King used pleasant, natural scents in therapy sessions in conjunction with such tension-reducing techniques as deep breathing, visualization, sound and heat. The patients learned to associate a particular fragrance with deep relaxation, and could later use the fragrance to draw on the association.

Positive programming with scent to relieve anxiety and stress has been around for a long time. In 12th-century Arabia, the Moslem doctor Al-Samarqandi wrote that breathing the fumes of the rose and sandalwood would "quiet the heat of brain." Myrrh and frankincense are also said to induce sleep and relaxation. The famous Egyptian fragrance *kyphi*, a perfume of frankincense, myrrh, calamus and spikenard, was used to encourage sleep, alleviate anxieties and brighten dreams. To ease migraine headaches, Al-Samarqandi suggested sniffing violets.

The use of sedative fragrances remained a part of health care into the 19th century, when Dr. W. S. Watson found that certain scents, especially rose, sedated mental patients. Attar of rose appeared in a 19th-century medical journal as a remedy for "nervous digestion." In 1954, Austrian perfumer Dr. Paul Jellinek classified rose as a "narcotic" scent.

In the early 1920s, Italian doctors G. Gatti and R. Cayola concluded that "the sense of smell has, by reflex action, an enormous influence on the function of the central nervous system" after extensive experiments showed that certain smells relaxed psychologically disturbed patients. When these essential oils were inhaled (or ingested), pulse rate, blood circulation and breathing changed. Most sedating were the citrus scents melissa, neroli and petitgrain, along with chamomile, asafetida, valerian and opopanax. Gatti and Cayola observed that where repeated or increased doses resulted in sedation, light initial doses were often experienced as stimulating.

When Dr. Henry D. Walter and his associates started to record the brain waves called "contingent negative variation" (CNV) in the 1960s, they found that such waves surged whenever a person looked forward to an event or ingested a stimulant such as coffee. When the subject felt drowsy or took a sedative drug, production of these brain waves was reduced. Fragrance also affected CNV brain waves, but unlike coffee or drugs, produced no change in heart rate, reaction time or alertness. The most sedative scents (in order of effectiveness) were lavender, bergamot, marjoram, sandalwood, lemon and chamomile—some of the same ones noted by Al-Samarqandi and, later, by Gatti and Cayola. Modern-day aromatherapists regard these scents as among the most emotion-balancing, specifically helpful in the treatment of depression, anxiety, headaches and strain from overwork.

STIMULATION

Workers at Tokyo's Kajima and Shimizu construction companies, and at Idemitsu Oil Development Company, are experiencing aromatherapy benefits firsthand. Throughout their work day, they are kept alert by fragrances regulated by a computer-controlled air-conditioning system. At Kajima, lemon is the morning wake-up call, followed by rose, which has employees working contentedly through the late morning. After lunch, an invigorating waft of cypress keeps workers awake. Shimizu disperses lavender and peppermint into offices and conference rooms to set a positive mood, boost work efficiency, and dispel physical drowsiness and mental fatigue. Lounges and restrooms are scented with cinnamon, and the hotel lobby contains a refreshing lemon. (Shimizu claims that scented air even reduces the urge to smoke.) On the way home, employees can stop off downtown at one of several atomizer-equipped phone booths for an aromatherapy escape from the stress of commuter traffic.

Dr. Henry D. Walter's studies on CNV brain-wave patterns identified peppermint, clove, basil and ylang-ylang as stimulants, as well as the somewhat weaker rose, patchouli, lemongrass and sage. Researchers determined that these oils arouse the autonomic nervous system, which controls such involuntary activities as breathing and blood pressure. This prevents the sharp drop in sustained attention that typically occurs after 30 minutes of work, sometimes even earlier. Adding physiological stress, such as adrenal overactivity, strain and/or boredom, to the workload can result in drowsiness, irritability and headaches.

To test the effects of fragrance on alertness and stress, researchers William N. Dember and Joel S. Warm gave subjects at the University of Cincinnati the difficult and stressful task of identifying patterns of lines on a computer for 40 minutes. Those working in rooms scented with lily-of-the-valley, benzoin, spiced-apple, forest, sandalwood or peppermint showed the best performance: 88 percent correct answers, compared to 65 percent from those in the unscented rooms. Interestingly, when questioned later most of the members of the first group didn't believe that the fragrances had affected their performance.

Psychologists refer to the experience of smell stimulating memory as the "Marcel Proust phenomenon." When the French novelist dipped a biscuit in his tea, the aroma brought back the flood of childhood memories that formed the basis of his multi-volume masterwork, *Remembrance of Things Past*. Certainly, we've all had at least one experience in which an aroma has brought back long-forgotten but still distinct memories. In fact, scientists tell us that our memory retention is much stronger when linked to smell than to sight. Researcher Trygg Engen of Brown University found that the memory recall associated with scent is at least twice that of visual recall. That's why a whiff of a certain perfume or some other fragrance that you haven't smelled for years will propel you back in time. With the scent comes everything associated with that aromatic experience: sights, sounds and emotional impressions.

In one study connecting the sense of smell with memory, 72 students smelled chocolate while they looked at a list of words and wrote down the corresponding antonyms. The next day, those who were given chocolate to smell again recalled an average of 21 percent of the words on the original list, while those deprived of chocolate averaged only 17 percent. Later studies showed the same results using unpleasant scents, such as the camphorous aroma of mothballs.

Fragrance has proved useful to therapists in encouraging patients to recall early memories and associated emotions. Psychologist André Virel encourages his clients to sniff vanilla in order to recall childhood memories. Perhaps unsurprisingly, he's found that pleasant odors tend to produce pleasant memories.

SCENT AND SOUL

Temple doors made out of sandalwood greet worshippers in India. Native Americans purify themselves with smudge sticks of cedar and sage. Heavy clouds of frankincense and myrrh fill Catholic churches on holy days. In the Mediterranean, and eventually throughout Europe, the fragrance of rosemary came to represent birth, death and transition. It was thrown on the casket when someone died, "for remembrance," and was also worn by brides. Rosemary was included in wedding ceremonies as a hint for the couple to remember their vows. It also served as a reminder of all the generations that had gone before—and those that would spring forth from the new union.

In most ancient cultures, the perfume industry was in the hands of the priests, with perfume workshops located in the temple. Incense served as a medium or pathway through which human prayers reached the gods. With incense the "soul" of the plant—that is, the essential oil—was called upon to raise the soul of the worshipper. Essential oils also represented the potential of the soul to find release from the material world. The Biblical prophet Isaiah, for example, speaks of the "soul" of perfume boxes carried by the "daughters of Zion."

Many religious fragrances originate in tree sap, regarded, along with blood, as a carrier of a regenerative "life force." Because the ancients felt a special reverence for trees—regarding them as a link between earth and sky, the mundane and the eternal—the sweet smell of burning sap amounted to an evocation of the divine nature.

Rich with symbolism, the history of aromatherapy has long been tied in with spiritual beliefs. Psychologist Dwight Hine concurs that odors create "an emotional, ecstatic state of consciousness that [renders] individuals more susceptible to religious experience." Danish psychotherapist Arne Meander uses aromatherapy to help patients regain their spiritual awareness and put them back in touch with their own healing powers.

PART II

Therapy

The smell of violets hidden in the green
Pour'd back into my empty soul and frame
The times when I remember to have been
Joyful and free from blame

—Alfred Lord Tennyson

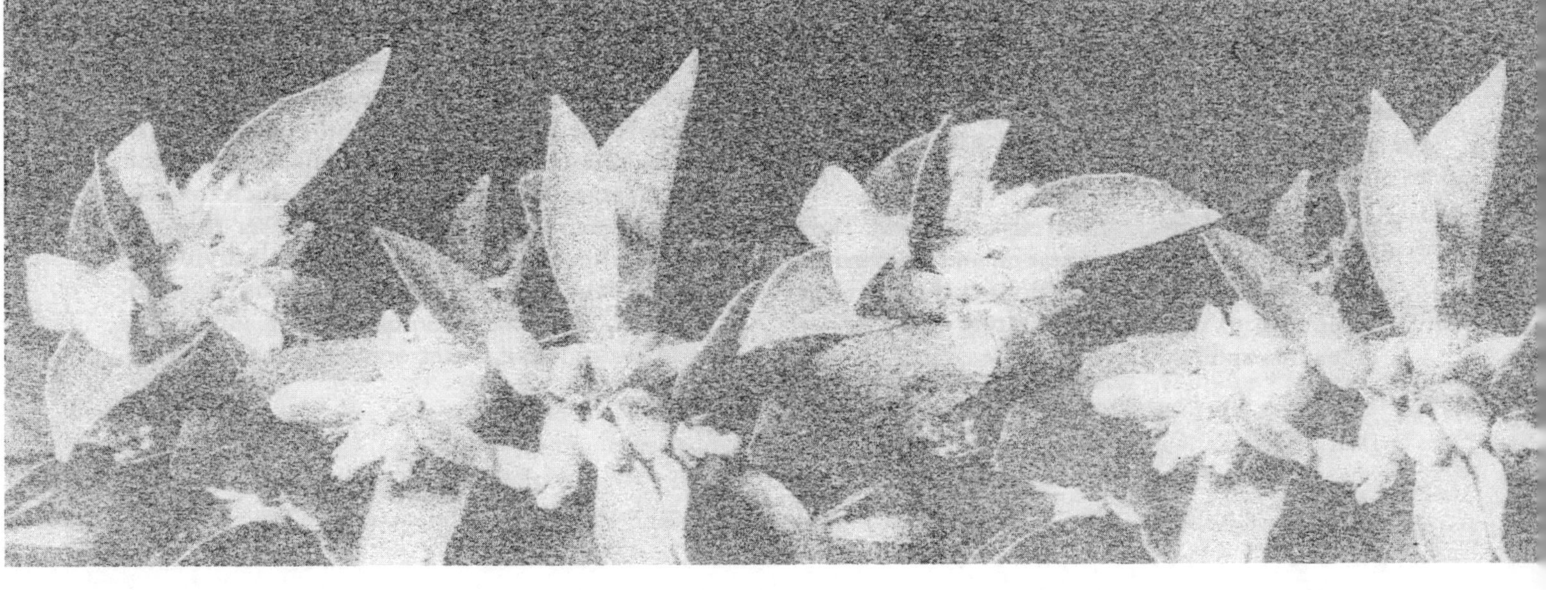

4

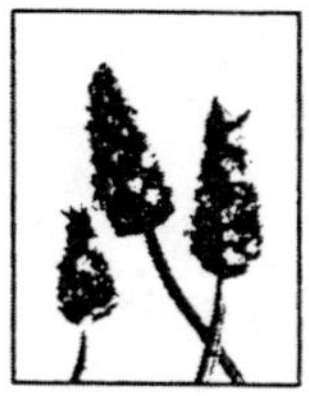

Guidelines for Using Essential Oils and Herbs

Essential oils are very versatile and can be used in a number of ways. To use them effectively, however, you need to be aware of safety issues, recommended dilutions and methods of application. This chapter will also introduce you to the different ways in which herbal preparations can be combined with aromatherapy treatments, as well as to the different carrier oils from which you may choose. Always keep a meticulous record of how you make your herbal preparations. Your notes should include ingredients and proportions, the date you started and completed the preparation, processing procedures, comments, improvements to be made next time. Label finished products with the date the product was made, ingredients and instructions for use.

SAFETY PRECAUTIONS

Because essential oils are concentrated, highly potent substances, a working knowledge of how to use them safely is vital to the success of your efforts. The potential hazards of an essential oil depend on the compounds in the oil, the dosage and frequency used, and the method of application. Here are a few guidelines to ensure safe and effective use of essential oils:

- Don't use undiluted essential oils on the skin. They can cause burning, skin irritation and photosensitivity. There are a few exceptions to this rule: it is acceptable to use the nonirritating oils lavender or tea tree undiluted on burns, insect bites, pimples and other skin eruptions—as long as you don't have extremely sensitive skin. If you find an essential oil irritating but would like to use it, and have determined that the irritation is not due to an allergy, try massaging the diluted blend into the soles of your feet. The oil will not irritate the skin, and will still enter the body.
- Use only pure essential oils from plants.
- Test for sensitivities. Most people with sensitivities to synthetic fragrances are not sensitive to high-quality essential oils. Also people who are allergic to, say, chamomile tea will not necessarily be allergic to the essential oil. If you are uncertain about an oil, do a *patch test* of a 2-percent dilution in the crook of the arm or on the back of the neck at the hairline. Twelve hours is ample time for a reaction to occur. If redness or itching develops, you may want to try a less potent dilution, or choose an appropriate substitute for the irritating oil.
- Use with caution those essential oils that result in photosensitivity. Citrus oils can irritate skin, and some of them will cause uneven pigmentation of the skin upon exposure to sun lamps or sunlight. This is especially true of bergamot, which contains bergaptene, a powerful photosensitizer that will cause allergic reactions in some individuals. (Bergaptene-free oil is available.) Of the citrus oils, bergamot is the most photosensitizing, followed by cold-pressed lime, bitter orange, and to some de-

gree, lemon and grapefruit. Of the lemon oils, California oil is the least photosensitizing. If you are using photosensitizing oils on your skin, do so at night, stay indoors, or wait at least four hours before exposing your skin to ultraviolet light.

- Use with caution those essential oils that are irritating to mucous membrane (the lining of the digestive, respiratory and genito-urinary tracts) and skin. Keep all essential oils away from the eyes.
- Keep all essential oils out of the reach of young children; older children can be taught to respect and properly use essential oils, but they should nevertheless be supervised. In general, when treating children with essential oils use one-third to one-half the adult dosage and select only nontoxic oils. Among the best and safest essential oils for children are lavender, tangerine, mandarin, neroli, frankincense, petitgrain and Roman chamomile.
- Vary the essential oils you use. Using the same facial oil blend for a long period of time is acceptable because it covers a very small part of the body, but daily application of the same blend of oils over your entire body for more than two weeks is not recommended. It is wise to alternate with a blend of different oils containing different chemical constituents at least every two weeks. Uninterrupted use of some oils exposes your liver and kidneys to chemical constituents that may be harmful over time. Rotating the oils gives your body time to process them and allows each oil to work on different levels in its own unique way.
- Don't take essential oils orally for therapeutic purposes. Safe ingestion of oils requires a great deal of training and is therefore not recommended for beginners. The exception is when we suggest using essential oils to flavor foods (see Chapter 10: Essential Oils in the Kitchen). The dosages per serving in these recipes are minimal and harmless.
- Use essential oils cautiously with those who are elderly, convalescing, or have serious health problems such as asthma, epilepsy or heart disease.
- Be cautious about using essential oils during pregnancy, especially during the first trimester. Even oils that are generally safe during this time may be too stimulating for women who are prone to miscarriage. Because so many oils are best avoided in pregnancy, it is easier to list the safe ones: gentle floral oils such as rose, neroli, lavender, ylang-ylang, chamomile and jasmine absolute, as well as the citruses, geranium, sandalwood, spearmint and frankincense.
- Overexposure to an essential oil, either through the skin or through inhalation, may result in nausea, headache, skin irritation, emotional unease or a "spaced-out" feeling. Getting some fresh air will help overcome these symptoms. If you ever experience skin irritation or accidentally get essential oils in the eyes, dilute with straight vegetable oil, not water.
- The following information is adapted from *The Essential Oil Safety Data Manual* by Robert Tisserand. We recommend this book to anyone interested in a thorough study of toxic oils.

Photosensitizing Essential Oils

angelica	lime
bergamot	opoponax
bitter orange	rue
cumin	verbena
lemon	

Mucous-Membrane Irritants

allspice	savory
cinnamon	spearmint
clove	thyme (except linalol)
oregano	

Skin Irritants

cinnamon	pimento
clove	savory
dwarf pine	thyme (except linalol)
oregano	wintergreen

Potentially Toxic Oils

Some of the oils in the following list have limited use externally; others are used for perfumery. We have included Latin names to avoid any confusion.

almond, bitter (*Prunus amygdalus* var. *amara*)
inula (*Inula graveolens*)
khella (*Ammi visnaga*)
mugwort (*Artemesia vulgaris*)
pennyroyal (*Mentha pelugium*)
sassafras (*Sassafras albidum*)
thuja (*Thuja occidentalis*)
wintergreen (*Gaultheria procumbens*)

Very Toxic Essential Oils

We recommend not using the following oils at all.

ajowan (*Ptychotis ajowan, Carum ajowan*)
arnica (*Arnica montana*)
boldo (*Peumus boldus*)
buchu (*Barosma betulina*)
calamus (*Acorus calamus*)
cascarilla (*Croton eluteria*)
chervil (*Anthriscus cerefolium*)
camphor, brown and yellow (*Cinnamomun camphora*)
deer tongue (*Carphephorus odoratissimus*)
horseradish (*Cochlearia armoracia, Armoracia rusticana*)
jaborandi (*Pilocarpus jaborandi*)
mustard (*Brassica nigra*)
narcissus (*Narcissus poeticus*)
nutmeg (*Myristica fragrans*)
parsley (*Petroselinum sativum, Carum sativum*)
rue (*Ruta graveolens*)
santolina (*Santolina chamaecyparissus*)
Spanish broom (*Spartium junceum*)
tansy (*Tanacetum vulgare*)
tonka (*Dipteryx odorata*)
turmeric (*Curcuma longa*)
wormseed (*Chenopodium ambrosioides, C. anthelminticum*)
wormwood (*Artemisia absinthium*)

METHODS OF APPLICATION

Dilutions

The most effective way to dilute essential oils is in a carrier oil. A carrier can be any high-quality vegetable oil, such as almond, apricot, hazelnut, olive, grapeseed or sesame.

A safe and effective dilution for most aromatherapy applications is 2 percent, which translates to 2 drops of essential oil per 100 drops of carrier oil. There is no need to go beyond a 3-percent dilution for any purpose. In aromatherapy, more is not better; in fact, "more" may cause adverse reactions. Some oils, such as lavender, are sedating in low dilutions and stimulating in high dilutions. A 1-percent dilution should be used on children, pregnant women, the elderly and those with health concerns.

You can create a safe and effective remedy with just one, two or three oils. When combining essential oils in a therapeutic blend, it is best for beginners to keep it simple, using no more than five oils at a time. Using more than five may lead to unpredictable results because of the complex chemistry created by the combination of all the oils.

1% dilution:	5-6 drops essential oil per ounce of carrier oil
2% dilution:	10-12 drops essential oil per ounce of carrier oil
3% dilution:	15-18 drops essential oil per ounce of carrier oil

We are often asked, "How big is a drop?" This is a very good question, because the size of a drop varies depending on the size of the dropper opening, as well as on the temperature and the viscosity (thickness) of the essential oil. A drugstore dropper will probably be accurate enough for your purposes.

Some people find it easier to use drops; others prefer measuring their essential oils by the teaspoon. Teaspoons are usually more convenient when preparing large quantities. Whatever your preference, use the chart on the following page as a general guideline. We've rounded off the measurements for your convenience. The ratios of drops to teaspoon were calculated using water, which has a medium viscosity compared with the range of viscosities found in essential oils.

Storage and Shelf Life

Store essential oils away from heat and light to preserve their freshness and potency. When stored prop-

Measurement Conversion Chart

10 drops	1/10 tsp.	1/60 oz.	about 1/8 dram	about 1/2 ml.
12.5 drops	1/8 tsp.	1/48 oz.	1/6 dram	about 5/8 ml.
25 drops	1/4 tsp.	1/24 oz.	1/3 dram	about 1 1/4 ml.
50 drops	1/2 tsp.	1/12 oz.	2/3 dram	about 2 1/2 ml.
100 drops	1 tsp.	1/6 oz.	1 1/3 dram	about 5 ml.
150 drops	1 1/2 tsp.	1/4 oz.	2 drams	about 13.5 ml.
300 drops	3 tsp.	1/2 oz.	4 drams	about 15 ml.
600 drops	6 tsp.	1 oz.	8 drams	about 30 ml.
24 teaspoons	(8 tablespoons)	4 oz.	1/2 cup	
48 teaspoons	(16 tablespoons)	8 oz.	1 cup	1/2 pint
96 teaspoons	(32 tablespoons)	16 oz.	2 cups	1 pint

erly, they have a shelf life of several years. The citrus oils have the shortest shelf life of all essential oils and are best used within one year. The longest-lasting oils, which improve as they age, tend to be the thick resins such as frankincense and myrrh, woods such as sandalwood, roots like vetiver, as well as other oils, including spikenard and patchouli.

Carrier oils should be stored away from heat and light to ensure their freshness. The addition of jojoba oil as 10 percent of your carrier oil will help extend the shelf life of your blend by slowing down oxidation that leads to rancidity. Vitamin E oil is an excellent antioxidant; adding it to any aromatherapy blend will help extend the life of most vegetable oils. One or two capsules (200-400 IU) per two-ounce bottle of carrier oil is enough. It is recommended that you make only enough of a blend to last a few months. A refrigerated blend may keep six months or more. Refrigeration of all vegetable oils is highly recommended.

Methods of Application at a Glance

Essential oils are versatile and effective in treating many common problems. The following guidelines are suitable for a single essential oil or a combination of oils. Many problems are best treated by a combination of methods. For example, a cold may be treated with an inhalant, a bath, a chest rub and a compress. Details on specific applications are presented throughout this book in the chapters on Facial Care, Massage and Therapeutics.

Suggested Dilutions for Various Methods of Application

Massage/Body Oil
2-3% dilution (10-12 drops per ounce of vegetable oil)
1% for pregnant women, people with health concerns, and children (5 drops per ounce of vegetable oil)

Bath
3-15 drops per tub, depending on the oil

Compress
5 drops per cup of water

Inhalant
3-5 drops in a bowl of hot water
Caution: never do an inhalation during an asthma attack.

Douche
3-5 drops per quart of warm water
Caution: Choose nonirritant oils only (e.g., lavender or tea tree).

Foot or Hand Bath
5-10 drops per quart of water

Sitz Bath
5-10 drops per sitz bath

Fragrant Body Water
5-10 drops per 4 ounces of water

Room Spray
20 drops per 4 ounces of water

Gargle or Mouthwash
1-2 drops per 1/4 cup of water

Liniment
3% dilution

Carrier Oils

Vegetable oils high in vitamins A, E and F—soothing, skin-softening, nourishing and rich in nutrients that enrich the skin—are among the best carriers of essential oils. They are called *fixed oils* because their large molecules stay in the plant instead of being easily released, as are the essential oils. This means that they are often extracted with heat or solvent-extracted (a process that also uses heat to extract the solvent). The one exception is olive oil, which can be cold-pressed, although less oil is obtained with this method, resulting in a more expensive product. Whenever possible, choose vegetable oils that are expeller-pressed or cold-pressed, which means they have not been exposed to temperatures over 110 degrees.

Unlike essential oils, vegetable oil molecules are large and do not easily penetrate the skin, making them an ideal medium for cosmetic products. The "saturation rate" of carrier oils measures how thick they are. The more saturated the oil, the thicker it is, the longer it stays on the skin, and the longer its shelf life. On the other hand, unsaturated oils give the illusion that they are being absorbed into the skin when they are actually evaporating. The most suitable oil depends on the application. Most body workers prefer saturated oil for massage, but many cosmetics use less saturated oils that feel less thick and sticky.

Other factors to consider are smell and color. The light smell and color of almond, hazelnut and grapeseed oils put them among the most preferred oils for cosmetics. (We've found that you need to go easy on using unrefined oils, which can leave you smelling like food).

Characteristics of Common Carrier Oils

Almond—Almond is an affordable, nourishing oil, well suited for massage. It provides just the right slip and glide, without wasting oil.

Apricot—This oil is derived from the kernel of the apricot pit. Its cost is comparable to that of almond, but it has a lighter consistency. Suitable for body oils and lotions.

Avocado—Deep green with lots of skin-nourishing vitamins, this thick oil is very rich on its own but combines nicely with other oils. It is well suited for dry-skin conditions.

Borage, Evening Primrose, Black Currant—The oils in this group are high in gamma linoleic acid (GLA), an important fatty acid that helps maintain healthy skin and repair skin damaged by the sun. Their rejuvenating effects are especially useful for treating mature skin. These oils can be used sparingly in a carrier blend (10 percent); because they are expensive, price alone will probably keep you from using too much.

Castor—Castor oil is very viscous and not normally used in aromatherapy, although it may be added in small amounts to formulas for eczema or other dry-skin conditions. Herbalists use castor oil to make compresses that break down fibrous tissue, enhance immunity and detoxify the liver. Sulfated castor oil is water-soluble and often used for aromatherapy bath oils.

Caulophyllum Inophyllum—This is a native of tropical Asia and was used in many Polynesian islands, and considered sacred. Known as *kamanu* or *kamani* in Hawaii, *tamanu* in the South Seas and *'fetau* in Samoa (Another variety, "faraha," is from Madagascar.), it is nontoxic and nonirritating, but rather expensive and thick, so you may want to combine it with another carrier oil. Anti-inflammatory and pain-relieving properties make Caulophyllum suitable for sciatica, rheumatism and shingles. It is antibacterial and nonirritating to mucous membranes and can be used to treat vaginitis and cervical erosion, infected wounds, eczema, psoriasis, chapped skin, cracked nipples, chemical or heat burns, and anal fissures. Historically, it was used extensively to treat leprosy.

Cocoa butter—Similar to coconut oil in consistency, cocoa butter is derived from cocoa beans and has a distinctive "chocolate" scent. It will overpower the odor of most essential oils, but may be used in small proportions as a thickener in lotions and creams. When combined with neroli, the fragrance is reminiscent of an exotic, delectable dessert.

Coconut—Highest in saturated fats, coconut oil is solid at room temperature. (It is twice as saturated as lard.) It can be used in conjunction with other oils for massage, and in body lotion or cream recipes. Although coconut oil has a long history of use in many tropical countries, it is often solvent-extracted, and if so, is not recommended for use on the face; it can cause allergic reaction in sensitive individuals.

Corn—The oil comes from our familiar table corn, mostly from the germ found in the corn's kernel. This oil is quite stable because it contains a large amount of vitamin E, which prevents oxidation. Corn-germ oil is also available, but has a strong odor.

Grapeseed—Light in texture, this odorless oil is mildly astringent and useful for acne or oily skin. Unfortunately, the seed is always solvent-extracted and is unavailable cold-pressed, causing sensitivity in some individuals.

Hazelnut—Light and mildly fragranced, this easily absorbed oil is useful in facial blends for those with a tendency toward oily skin. Hazelnut oil makes a great base for calendula infusions (see the section on herb-infused oils) and for all cosmetic purposes, including massage.

Jojoba—The carrier of choice for perfumery, jojoba is technically not an oil but a liquid wax. It does not oxidize or become rancid. A small amount (10 percent) can be used to extend the shelf life of all blends. Because jojoba is very similar to the sebum produced by our own skin, it is particularly beneficial in facial and body oils, and it is also recommended for scalp and hair treatments. It is derived from the seed of the desert shrub.

Kukui—The thinnest, lightest oil for the face, kukui provides just the right amount of lubrication without leaving a greasy feeling. The kukui nut, native to Hawaii, is high in linoleic and linolenic acids, and is rapidly absorbed into the skin. It was used by the Hawaiians for skin conditioning after sun exposure (but is not a sunscreen). Kukui-nut oil has a low toxicity level, but it is laxative and therefore should not be ingested. It has a distinct odor and is very expensive, so you may want to combine it with other oils.

Macadamia—Slightly more viscous than kukui and also from Hawaii, macadamia oil is similar to both mink oil and sebum, our skin's own natural oil. Its lightness makes it ideal as a base for facial or hair-care products, and it combines well with kukui.

Olive—This oil is a favorite for dry skin, but the odor is a little strong for some people. It may be blended with other oils and has a nice texture for massage. This is one of the best mediums for herb-infused oils intended for medicinal applications, such as in salves or rectal or vaginal suppositories. Pure olive oil has excellent stability and can be stored without refrigeration for a year. (Greek olive oil is greener and more acidic than oil from Italy or California.)

Rice Bran—This oil is naturally high in mixed tocopherols (vitamin E) and ferulic acid, another natural antioxidant. It flows on smoothly and is moderately penetrating without being greasy or sticky. Good for massage or lotions.

Rosehip seed—Another oil high in GLA, pungent rosehip seed is the very best for regenerative skin care. It is rich and expensive, so we recommend blending it with other oils (10-20 percent rosehip-seed oil in carrier blend). Combine with infused calendula oil to treat stretch marks, burns or scars.

Safflower—This oil comes from an herb that is cultivated in California and Arizona, where it turns fields aglow with its colorful flowers. Safflower oxidizes easily, especially the natural oil. It can be used in massage blends.

Sesame Seed—This oil contains sesomoline, a natural preservative. Sesame has long been used in Ayurvedic medicinal preparations and is said to be rejuvenating. The unrefined variety has a strong scent, which is the biggest drawback to using this oil alone as a carrier. Good as a base for herb preparations.

Soybean—First introduced from the Orient to the United States, this oil was rarely used before 1950. It now accounts for more than 65 percent of all oil used commercially in the United States. Because of its low oil content (16-18 percent), it is often solvent-extracted. Soybean oil is high in linoleic acid and susceptible to oxidation. Use as a part of a massage blend.

Squalene—Vegetable sources of this oil product are olive, wheat germ and rice bran oils. Squalene can also be derived from shark liver oil. It is used as a fixative in perfumes and as a bactericide, and is very expensive; 5-10 percent in a carrier blend is sufficient. Human sebum is 25 percent squalene.

Wheat germ—Too thick and rich on its own, this oil is a useful addition to any carrier blend. It is high in vitamin B, and because it contains the antioxidant vitamins A and E, it will help extend the shelf life of your blends. Add 10 percent to your carrier-oil blend.

Vegetable Oils

The more saturated an oil, the thicker its consistency and the longer it can be stored without refrigeration. Also, the lower the iodine value, the better the oil will keep. Values can vary according to the source of the oil. Some oils also contain other ingredients that improve their preservation, such as sesame oil.

Oil	% of Saturated Fats	Iodine Value
Coconut	91	9
Cocoa Butter	50	40
Olive	20	84
Peanut	20	92
Rice	17	104
Corn	17	124
Wheat Germ	18	125
Walnut	16	138
Soy	15	130
Sesame	13	110
Almond	5-10	100
Apricot	5-10	100
Sunflower	6-8	130
Safflower	6	143
Castor	3	84

The values are based on information from *Bailey's Industrial Oil and Fat Products,* edited by Daniel Swern, and *Food Oils and Their Uses,* by Theodore J. Weiss, USDA research chemist.

HERBAL PREPARATIONS

Never pass up the opportunity to use herbs in your aromatherapy formulations. When the essential oil of a plant is deemed too strong for a particular person or application, the herb itself in tea or tincture form is likely a safe and effective substitute. When used together, whole plants and essential oils often create a synergy with greater potential for healing than either used alone.

Herb quality is as important to herbalism as purity of essential oils is to aromatherapy. Growing your own herbs is ideal, but we realize that many of you will be buying herbs from an herb or natural-food store. The good news is that it is much easier to determine good herb quality by smelling, seeing and tasting than it is with essential oils. Dried herbs should not be brown and lifeless; they should be fragrant, colorful and, ideally, organically grown or responsibly picked in the wild. Buying direct from the grower, wildcrafter (one who picks wild herbs), or local sources such as farmers' markets, where you can inquire about growing methods, is probably the next best thing to growing your own herbs.

The following recipes provide a useful basis for making basic herbal preparations. They can be made either with individual herbs ("simples") or a combination of herbs ("compounds"). So get creative! If you need more detailed information on the specific uses of individual herbs, consult a good herb book such as Kathi's *Herbs, an Illustrated Encyclopedia* (Friedman/Fairfax).

Preparing Herb-Infused Oils

Oils made by macerating (steeping) herbs in vegetable oil are called *infused oils.* The oils can be used instead of plain carrier oils in all of your aromatherapy preparations.

Finely chop (or coarsely grind) one cup dried herbs in a blender. Place the herbs in a wide-mouth jar and add enough oil to cover. Check the mixture in a day or two; you may need to add a bit more oil. Keep the mixture in a warm place and shake daily. The ideal temperature is 70-80 degrees Fahrenheit, but fluctuations in temperature will not harm the oil. Let the mixture steep for one week; by this time, the oil should have taken on the color, aroma and healing properties of the herb.

Strain the oil through a kitchen strainer, or through cheesecloth, muslin or a thin dishcloth. Most of the oil will drain out. To get every precious drop, press with the back of a spoon or wring out as much oil as possible. Compost the herbs and store the infused oil in a cool place.

There are many variations on this preparation. Choose a vegetable oil such as olive for medicinal preparations such as salves; choose hazelnut or another light oil for cosmetic applications or massage. It is difficult to give exact measurements for each herb, because they are different in texture, weight and volume. To double the strength, you can add a new batch of dried herb to the same oil. This is called a *double infusion.*

Another way to make infused oils is on the stove top. Place the dried herbs in a pot and cover them with oil. Gently warm the herb mixture over low heat (about 100° F) without a lid, stirring occasionally. (Be careful not to deep-fry your herbs.) After about six hours, strain, cool and bottle.

Some people like to use fresh herbs, although the water in fresh plants may cause the oil to mold and spoil. However, some oils—St. John's wort for example—must be made fresh. Wilt the plant material overnight to eliminate some of the water, then finely chop or crush them. Process as instructed above for dry herbs. Be sure that all the plant material is submerged and that there are no air bubbles.

When straining the oil, simply let the mixture drip; wringing or pressing will give you more oil, but also more water. When the water from the fresh plant has settled in the bottom of the jar, pour the oil off the top and discard the water. (Be prepared to lose a little oil.)

Don't confine yourself to making only medicinal or cosmetic oils. Experiment with creating culinary oils, too. Try a combination of basil, oregano, rosemary and garlic infused in olive oil. It's great on pasta or french bread!

Always keep a meticulous record of how you make your herbal preparations. Your notes should include ingredients and proportions, the date you started and completed the preparation, processing procedures, comments, and possible improvements to be made next time. Label finished products with the date the product was made, ingredients, and instructions for use.

Further Examples of Herb-Infused Oils

Alkanet—This is an infusion of alkanet root in vegetable oil. Because of its brilliant color, it is used as a pink coloring for cosmetic preparations.

Calendula—Very healing to the skin in all cosmetic applications, calendula is specifically recommended for burns and is also antimicrobial, making it suitable for the treatment of many types of skin infections. There is also a carbon-dioxide extract of calendula which is very concentrated and tarlike. It can be diluted in vegetable oil and added to any essential oil preparation.

Neem—Derived from a tree native to India, neem is used to treat a number of skin diseases, as an astringent, antibacterial and antiviral. It is also a preservative. The oil has a long history of use in treatment of hair loss, dandruff, excess sebum production, brittle nails, nail fungus and gum infections. This herb is hard to find unless you have a neem tree, but pre-prepared oil can be purchased.

St. John's Wort—Excellent for bruises, inflammation and nerve damage, St. John's wort is made from fresh flowering tops of the plant to obtain the desired deep red oil, high in the healing constituent hypericin.

Yarrow—For treating the genito-urinary system (see Chapter 5: Therapeutics).

Herbal Boluses

Herbal boluses are vaginal or rectal suppositories used to treat chronic infections, nonspecific vaginitis, cysts, and hemorrhoids. See "Reproductive System."

Ingredients: 1/8 cup finely powdered herbs
1/4 cup cocoa butter
15-20 drops appropriate essential oil

Melt the cocoa butter over low heat and add the finely powdered herbs to form a thick, pliable paste. Add the essential oil. Drop the mixture by the teaspoonful onto a cold plate and form into a suppository shape about the size of your little finger (or you can mold it into a long, thin roll). Refrigerate until firm. Remove the hardened mixture and cut it with a warm knife into 1 1/2-inch lengths. Date and store boluses in glass or plastic in the refrigerator.

For treatment, insert one bolus each evening for seven days. Women may want to wear a panty liner and gently douche every couple of days.

Herbal Salves

Ingredients: 1 cup herb-infused oil
3/4 ounce beeswax, shaved

Warm the herb-infused oil in a pan and add the beeswax. (More beeswax will create a salve with a firmer consistency, which won't melt in hot temperatures.) You can shave the beeswax with a wide-hole cheese grater. (For a quick cleanup; heat the grater over the kitchen stove and wipe with paper towels.) Add essential oils at the end, after the salves cool a bit so that the oils do not evaporate. (You can also add the essential oils to the individual jars before pouring.)

Lip balms are made the same way as salves, but use 1 ounce beeswax.

Herb Tea: Infusions and Decoctions

For infusions, pour boiling water over fresh or dried herbs, let them steep while covered for 5-10 minutes, strain and drink. Cover steeping herbs to keep in the precious volatile oils.

Infusions are good for delicate plant parts such as leaves, blossoms and fruits, or seeds and roots that are high in volatile oils. The amount of herb varies, but the general rule is one teaspoon dried herb, or one tablespoon fresh herb, per cup of water.

For hard plant parts, such as roots, barks, twigs and some seeds, decoctions are preferable. We prefer to soak the herbs in cold water overnight, bring the water and herbs to a boil, then lower the heat and simmer, covered, for at least 15 minutes. Roots and seeds that are high in volatile oils, such as ginger and valerian roots, or fennel and anise seeds, should be infused.

To make tea with both leaves and roots, start by soaking the herbs overnight in the refrigerator, then bring to a boil, remove from the heat and steep for 15 minutes. You can also decoct the roots first, remove from heat, add the leaves to the decoction and steep.

Teas are a great addition to bath water, especially for those with highly sensitive skin. Almost any herb or essential oil, alone or in combination, will do. Refrigerator storage is acceptable for up to three days.

Herbal Tinctures

Ingredients: dry or fresh herbs
vodka to cover

Chop or grind herbs before tincturing to expose more surface area of the plant to the vodka which contains only water and alcohol and is used to break down the plant matter and extract its qualities. Put the herbs in a jar with a tight-fitting lid and cover with menstruum. The proportion of herb to vodka is hard to specify, because the weight-to-volume of each herb varies so much. Make sure that the herb is completely covered. Check in a few days in case you need to add more vodka. Cover the jar tightly and let the herbs soak for two weeks in a cool, dark place, shaking daily, then strain. You'll be surprised to find how easy this is, and it costs much less than commercial tinctures.

Tinctures are best made with single herbs, and can then be mixed together to make compounds or formulas. This helps avoid undesirable constituent interactions that can occur when herbs are tinctured together. It also allows for more flexibility in blending tinctures into different combinations. Tinctures are taken orally, typically 15 to 30 drops three times a day, mixed in a little water or juice. One advantage herbal tinctures have over teas is that they need no refrigeration and remain potent for many years, take up little storage space, and are fast and easy to use, fitting into any busy lifestyle. They are also quickly and easily absorbed by the body.

Herbal Vinegars

Ingredients: fresh or dried herbs
vinegar to cover

Make sure the fresh or dried herbs are covered by the vinegar. Shake daily for two weeks, strain. Add essential oils to the vinegar after straining, but remember to shake well before use—essential oils do not mix with a watery carrier. These vinegars can be used to make "Queen of Hungary's water," other facial toners, hair rinses, baths, and douches. Vinegar also can be used as a substitute for alcohol in tincturing for those who are alcohol-intolerant, but it is not a good menstruum for extracting the resinous constituents contained in certain plants.

5

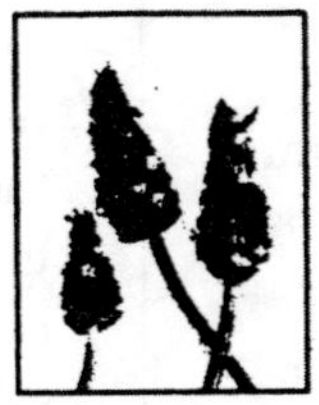

Therapeutics

In this chapter we explain how essential oils heal the body. We have divided the chapter into sections dealing with the major systems in the body—circulatory, digestive, respiratory, nervous, glandular, urinary, reproduction, dermal and musculoskeletal—as well as sections on ears and eyes, immunity and children. We suggest how to treat common ailments, things you would normally treat at home without the care of a doctor: the common cold; headache; a bout of indigestion; PMS; simple burns, bites and stings; muscular aches and pains. You may have formerly treated such disorders with over-the-counter drugs. The biochemical complexity of essential oils—most of which cannot be synthetically duplicated—allows them to act on many levels, and gives them multiple powers. You'll achieve not only health dividends, but also savings in your pocketbook.

As herbalists and aromatherapists, the authors of this book are eclectic in our approach to healing, using whatever remedy seems most appropriate. In some cases, we use aromatherapy exclusively; in others, we find that combining aromatherapy with herbs is more effective. To help you integrate the two modalities, we offer "herbal adjuncts," generally to be taken several times a day in teas, tinctures, capsules or tablets.

Because true holistic healing requires individual assessment and formation of a blend specific to each person, we do not give many recipes for specific ailments. We understand that some guidelines are needed, however, so to get you started we have given formula examples for general conditions in each section. Our goal is to give you the tools and confidence you need to develop your own blends as your understanding of working with essential oils increases. Refer to charts and the "Materia Medica" chapter.

Essential oils are extremely concentrated. Most of them are at least 50 times more potent than the herbs from which they are derived. In her book *Aromatherapy: The Complete Guide to Plant and Flower Essences for Health and Beauty*, Daniele Ryman states that one drop of essential oil often represents the potency of one ounce of plant material. This gives you an idea of their healing potential—and of the potential hazards of using essential oils improperly.

Only about 5 percent of the essential oils produced today are used in aromatherapy, but there are plenty from which to choose. In fact, if you become familiar with only 10 to 15 essential oils, you'll be able to treat many common problems. (It is better to know a few essential oils well than to know a little about many oils.)

Essential oils include muscle relaxants (marjoram and black pepper), digestive tonics (cardamom and mint), circulatory stimulants (rosemary and basil) and hormone precursors (clary sage and fennel). Many repair injured cells (lavender and helichrysum); others help carry away metabolic waste (grapefruit and juniper). In addition, a number of essential oils enhance immunity, working with the body to heal itself. They are capable of stimulating the production of phago-

Ten Basic Essential Oils

Lavender	overall first-aid oil; antiviral and antibacterial, boosts immunity, antidepressant, anti-inflammatory, antispasmodic
Chamomile	anti-inflammatory, antiallergenic, digestive, relaxant, antidepressant
Marjoram	antispasmodic, anti-inflammatory, antiseptic
Rosemary	stimulating to circulation, relieves pain, decongestant, improves circulation
Tea tree	antifungal, antiyeast, antibacterial
Cypress	astringent, stimulating to circulation, antiseptic, astringent
Peppermint	digestive, clears sinuses, antiseptic, decongestant, stimulant
Eucalyptus	decongestant, antiviral, antibacterial, stimulant
Bergamot	antidepressant, antiparasitic, anti-inflammatory
Geranium	balancing to mind and body, antifungal, anti-inflammatory

cytes (white blood cells that attack invaders), and some (e.g., tea tree and lavender) are antitoxic for insect bites and stings.

Many essential oils have been proven effective against fungi and yeast (tea tree, lavender and geranium), parasites (bergamot) and viruses (cinnamon, thyme and *Eucalyptus radiata*). Others fight infection with amazing effectiveness, killing bacteria by disrupting their life cycle. According to Dr. Jean-Claude Lapraz, M.D., a specialist in essential oils, most essential oils lower the pH of the blood slightly, creating an inhospitable environment for bacteria, which thrive in an alkaline environment.

Unlike conventional antibiotic drugs, which may cause undesirable side effects, essential oils are "probiotic": they not only kill pathogenic bacteria, but tend to leave beneficial bacteria (intestinal flora) intact. This seems an exclusive prerogative of natural healing and remains a mystery to science. Also, bacteria typically do not acquire a resistance to essential oils, as they so often do to antibiotic drugs.

Essential oils act quickly in the body. Some are detectable in the breath within minutes after application to the skin, and are eliminated from the body within several hours. Repeated applications may be required, especially when treating acute disorders that require keeping a constant level of essential oil active in the body.

Remember that less is more when it comes to aromatherapy. Consistent low doses are safest and most effective.

One advantage of aromatherapy treatments is that they don't need to work their way through the entire body to treat a particular area. Most of the essential oils suggested in this section are intended for dilution in a carrier oil. You can massage these diluted oils directly over the area that needs treatment—on the chest, for example, to treat congested lungs, or on the stomach in cases of indigestion. Application by inhalation or bath is also appropriate for many treatments.

Essential oils are perfectly safe when used in the suggested dilutions, although applications complicated by pregnancy, epilepsy, serious health problems and some medications do call for caution. A patch test is recommended before using any formula. (See Safety Precautions in the "Guidelines" chapter for further information on safety, applications, dilutions and carrier oils; also, please note the various "considerations" in the "Materia Medica" chapter.)

BODY SYSTEMS

Health and vitality depend on the harmonious and collective functioning of each organ in the body. Therefore, the identification and separation of systems and their association with various oils is a simplification, albeit a necessary one. Also, because most plants have multiple actions, many are listed below for more than one system or symptom.

Heart and Circulation

The circulatory system transports blood throughout the body. It includes the heart and the blood vessels, as well as the lymphatic system, which supplies nutrients and moves cellular fluid through the system, cleansing the body of waste. Lymph nodes located throughout the body—but particularly in the throat, groin, breasts and under the arms—act as centers for filtering the blood.

One of the best essential oils for a lymphatic massage is true bay (*Laurus nobilis*); lemon and grapefruit are also good. (A good carrier oil for these essential oils is calendula.) Use basil, rosemary, thyme, marjoram and clove to improve general circulation. Stress-related heart problems respond well to a sedating massage of melissa, neroli, lavender and ylang-ylang. Along with marjoram and ginger, these oils also help normalize high blood pressure. (Studies show that just sniffing neroli can lower high blood pressure.)

Chamomile, myrtle and cypress ease the inflammation and pain of varicose veins, phlebitis and hemorrhoids; frankincense constricts distended veins. All of these oils are especially effective in an infused oil of St. John's wort. If the skin is ulcerated and broken, apply a compress of carrot-seed essential oil. Soak a cloth in water to which a few drops of oil have been added, wring out, then place over area.

Formula for Varicose Veins

6 drops cypress
3 drops myrtle
3 drops German chamomile
2 drops frankincense (optional)
1 ounce St. John's wort oil

Combine ingredients. Apply externally. This can also be made into a salve by heating the oil and adding 1/2 teaspoon shaved beeswax before adding the essential oils.

Herbal Adjuncts—Among the herbs which strengthen heart and blood pressure are hawthorn flower and berry, and motherwort. Lymphatic cleaners include echinacea, cleavers and Oregon grape root, which may also be taken as teas, tinctures or pills.

The kitchen cupboard supplies many foods whose essential oils enhance circulation, make blood vessels more elastic and inhibit blood clotting. These include garlic, onion, cayenne and ginger. Ginger either raises blood pressure by restricting external blood flow, or lowers it by dilating surface blood vessels. Garlic and onions also lower high blood pressure. Lemongrass contains five different compounds that inhibit blood clotting.

Digestive System

Our health and vitality depend largely on how effectively we process and assimilate nutrients, as well as on how thoroughly we eliminate waste. What we eat is important, but so are how and when we eat. Creating a peaceful environment, eating fresh whole foods and proper elimination constitute a good start toward digestive harmony.

Aromas signal the brain that food is on the way, so simply sniffing a pleasant food aroma, such as pasta sauce or baking bread, begins a chain reaction that sets the stomach grumbling in anticipation. The response is almost immediate, as digestive fluids are released in the mouth, stomach and small intestine.

The essential oils found in common culinary herbs such as rosemary, basil, cumin, anise, coriander, ginger and cinnamon not only make food tasty, but help digestion. In addition, some spices have special applications: cumin relieves indigestion-promoted headaches, rosemary improves poor food absorption, and basil helps overcome nausea even from chemotherapy or radiation treatments, even when conventional anti-nausea drugs have had little effect. Lemongrass is used in Southeast Asia to relieve indigestion. To decrease appetite, try dill and fennel.

If you are plagued by ulcers or stomach acidity, try chamomile and sandalwood. Fennel seed and melissa relax the stomach muscles while soothing irritation and inflammation. Try a small amount of honey flavored with one of these oils in a cup of herb tea. (See the "Essential Oils in the Kitchen" chapter for instructions on how to make this honey.)

Poor digestion can also result from too little hydrochloric acid, which is needed to break down protein. Improperly digested protein is thought to be a cause of certain food allergies. Black pepper and juniper berry both increase stomach acid. Use these essential oils in a massage blend over the stomach, add fresh-ground pepper to your meal, or chew a couple of juniper berries before eating.

Ginger is one of the best remedies for nausea—especially motion and morning sickness—with peppermint running a close second. The British medical journal *Lancet* reported ginger more effective than the popular antihistamine drug Dramamine for preventing motion sickness, and unlike the drug ginger doesn't leave you feeling sluggish. These essential oils can be used in a 2-percent massage blend, although herb teas are both effective and tasty. Even eating ginger cookies, a piece of crystallized ginger (sold in Chinese food stores) or peppermint candy works.

Tummy Soother Massage Oil

5 drops chamomile
3 drops dill
2 drops ginger
2 drops peppermint
1 ounce carrier oil

Combine oils and gently massage the abdomen. For kids, use half the number of drops in the recipe.

Digestive Tonic Tea

1 teaspoon gingerroot
1/4 teaspoon cinnamon bark
1 teaspoon peppermint
1/2 teaspoon anise
1/4 teaspoon cardamom
3 cups water, boiling

Mix herbs together, pour water over them. Drink a cup 30 minutes after your meal. The hot water extracts the essential oils from the herbs.

Natural Ginger Ale

3 cups digestive tea (recipe above)
1/4 cup honey
1 cup carbonated water
1 lemon slice

Stir honey into warm tea. Add carbonated water and lemon just before serving.

Bowel Problems

The bowels can become irritated or infected by various foods. Even excitement or stress can agitate the bowels. Ginger, peppermint, fennel, coriander and dill help counter gas. Peppermint is specific for irritable-bowel syndrome. For constipation, use rosemary or black pepper. For diarrhea use cypress, cinnamon and myrrh.

Garlic is one of the best ways to eliminate worms for the whole family, including pets. Fresh garlic should be eaten in meals or taken in capsules. Rosemary, thyme, tea tree and chamomile kill many types of worms; chamomile also decreases the resulting intestinal inflammation. Researchers have discovered that all 42 components in the ginger oil used in East Africa to kill parasites will, in isolation, kill roundworms in the intestine. (Some of these compounds actually worked better in studies than the commonly prescribed piperazine-citrate preparations.) These oils can also be used in a massage over the abdomen area as part of a more inclusive treatment.

The liver is also involved in digestion, and its health affects the entire body.

Liver Tonic

3 drops each:
chamomile
lemon
carrot
helichrysum
1 ounce carrier oil

Any of these oils can also be used alone. Massage the oil over the liver, or use it in a bath.

Herbal Adjuncts—Use at least one aromatic herb with any remedy for diarrhea or constipation, to prevent intestinal cramping. Turn to herbal "bitters" such as gentian, Oregon grape root, barberry and dandelion root to treat long-term digestive problems such as chronic diarrhea, constipation, indigestion and certain food allergies. These bitter tonics are best taken before meals. Laxatives include the mild-acting yellow dock, or the stronger cascara bark and senna leaf. To treat diarrhea use a blackberry root tincture. For stomach ulcers or overacidity, use soothing slippery elm and marshmallow, antispasmodic chamomile and wild yam, the natural antacid meadowsweet, and licorice, which helps diminish ulcers.

To eliminate worms, eat raw carrots, garlic and pumpkin seeds, as well as fibrous vegetables. Also, restrict carbohydrates and milk products. (Worms thrive on their sugars.) Then flush everything out with an herbal laxative. Repeat the treatment in a week to kill any newly hatched parasites.

Respiratory System

Afflictions of the respiratory system include irritation and infection of the ears, nose and throat. Respiratory problems also may involve congestion, which can be decreased by inhaling rosemary (especially the verbenone type), hyssop (use var. *decumbens* only), tea tree, eucalyptus, lavender or peppermint. Cypress helps dry up a persistent runny nose, and peppermint, tea tree and eucalyptus reduce sinus infection. Anise and cypress help reduce coughing.

Many asthma sufferers wage a constant battle with low-level congestion. Don't use essential oils during an asthma attack, but between attacks try a chest rub of German chamomile, frankincense or lavender. The chamazulene in chamomile releases cortisone from the adrenals. During an asthma attack, give a bath or treat the feet with these oils. (Hyssop can also be used, but be careful to only use var. *decumbens*.)

Ninety percent of respiratory ailments are caused by viruses. Oils of thyme, rosemary, peppermint, ravensare, tea tree, eucalyptus, bergamot, black pepper, melissa and hyssop inhibit most flu viruses. Lemon and eucalyptus oils are effective against bacteria that cause staph, strep and pneumonia infections. A 2-percent dilution makes an effective antiseptic gargle or vapor steam.

Steam treatment carries essential oils directly to sinuses and lungs, and provides warm, moist air to help open nasal and bronchial passages. To do a steam, boil a pan of water, turn off the heat, cool 1 minute, add 3-6 drops of essential oils to the water, and use a towel to corral the steam around your head as you breathe deeply. Essential oils can also be used in many humidifiers, or as an ingredient in steamy hot bath water.

If steaming is impractical—at the office, say, or while traveling—inhale a tissue scented with the oils, or use a natural-products nasal inhaler. These are sold in natural food stores, or you can make your own:

Homemade Nasal Inhaler

2 drops eucalyptus
2 drops rosemary
1 drop peppermint
1 tablespoon rock salt

Place a few pieces of rock salt in a vial and add the oils. The salt will quickly absorb the oil. Inhale.

An aromatic diffuser—a glass piece (often hand-blown) connected to a small electrical compressor—disinfects the atmosphere by releasing droplets of essential oil as a cool, fine mist. One advantage to using a diffuser is that the essential oil vapor can be directed into the nose, throat or even ear passages. It can be turned on in a sickroom for 10 to 15 minutes every hour to clear airborne bacteria.

Do not use thick oils such as vetiver, sandalwood, vanilla, myrrh and benzoin in a diffuser unless they are diluted with a thin oil—such as the citruses, eucalyptus or rosemary—or mixed with alcohol. If oils sit too long in a diffuser, they oxidize and thicken. Also, expressed citrus oils often contain sediment that may clog a diffuser. To clean or unclog it, soak the glass unit in alcohol and unplug the opening with a pin or toothpick. Rinse and air dry.

Diluted essential oils can also be used as a throat spray through "nebulization." A nebulizer sprayer, with its long spout that reaches to the back of the throat, used to be a standard item in the home medicine cabinet. A perfume atomizer or spray bottle will work just as well.

If you don't have a diffuser, simply combine water and essential oils in a spray bottle. Studies show that a two-percent dilution of eucalyptus oil kills 70 percent of airborne staph bacteria.

Disinfectant Room Spray

3 drops eucalyptus
1 drop peppermint
2 drops pine
1 drop tea tree
2 drops bergamot
1 ounce of water

Combine ingredients. Shake well before using. The combination is also suitable as a chest rub. (Replace the water in this recipe with a carrier oil.)

Generations of Europeans, especially singers, have gargled sage, thyme or marjoram tea sweetened with honey to relieve laryngitis and tonsillitis. A few drops of essential oils diluted in two ounces of water may also do the trick. In case of sore throat, gargle frequently, at least every half-hour.

Throat Spray/Gargle

1/2 cup thyme or sage herb tea
3 drops each cypress, lemon, tea tree

Shake well to disperse the oils before each use. For a gargle, half a teaspoon of salt may be dissolved into the solution.

For lung congestion a salve or a massage oil containing essential oils can be rubbed over the chest, back and throat. The oils will be absorbed through the skin and lungs as the vapor is inhaled. Place a flannel fabric on the chest after rubbing in the oil to increase warmth. Commercial "vapor balms" still use derivatives of essential oils (or their synthetic-oil counterparts), such as thymol from thyme and menthol from mint, in a petroleum ointment base. Natural alternatives are also sold in natural-food stores.

Vapor Balm

2 teaspoons peppermint oil
3 teaspoons eucalyptus oil
1 teaspoon thyme oil (chemotype linalol is best)
1 cup olive oil
3/4 ounce beeswax

Melt beeswax into olive oil over very low heat. Cool a bit, add essential oils and stir. (Be sure to keep your face away from the oils as you stir them in.) Allow to harden. Store at room temperature.

Poultices are an age-old remedy for chest congestion. A ginger or onion compress on the chest breaks up lung congestion and makes breathing easier. Onions also help curb asthma and allergic reactions.

Poultice

1 onion, chopped and 1/4 cup ginger, grated
water

Lightly cook together in a little water until soft. Cool slightly, mash and apply to the chest while still warm. Cover with a soft cloth.

Herbal Adjuncts—Herbs that loosen mucus from the lungs include elecampane, horehound and mullein. Respiratory relaxants, such as wild cherry bark and wild lettuce, are used in cases of extreme spasmodic coughing. Demulcent herbs, which soothe inflamed mucous membranes, include flaxseed, marshmallow root and licorice. Use these herbs in a tea, tincture, pills or syrup.

Musculoskeletal System

Bones and muscles give form to the body and permit physical movement. Unless damaged by injury, the health of this system depends on the overall health of the body. With degenerative conditions such as arthritis and rheumatism, the entire body must be treated, especially the digestive and eliminative systems. Use anti-inflammatory essential oils that stimulate the circulation and eliminate toxins such as grapefruit, juniper and helichrysum. Pain relievers such as birch are also useful. A common sense diet—avoiding foods that create an acidic reaction, such as red meat, eggs and dairy foods—is also helpful. Refer to the "Massage" chapter for additional suggestions for the treatment of muscular aches and pains.

Some aromatherapists use rosemary and lemongrass to ease stiffness. According to Dr. Dietrich Gumbel, they remove lactic-acid buildup in the muscles. The following formula may also be used for arthritis.

Pain Formula

6 drops helichrysum
4 drops marjoram
2 drops juniper
4 drops birch or wintergreen
3 drops chamomile
3 drops lavender
3 drops ginger
2 ounces of carrier oil

Combine ingredients. This formula can be used in massage or bath.

Herbal Adjuncts—Anti-inflammatories include meadowsweet, willow bark and devil's claw, or cayenne, ginger, mustard and horseradish added to foods. Dandelion, sarsaparilla, burdock, celery seeds, parsley and yarrow help eliminate toxins through the kidneys. Pain relievers include valerian and St. John's wort.

Nervous System

The nervous system provides the intricate connection between mind and body. As a result of mental or emotional responses, a problem in one area of the body may affect another.

For stress in general, try bergamot, chamomile, lavender, melissa, clary sage, neroli, rose or jasmine. For insomnia due to mental agitation or overwork, clary sage, marjoram, ylang-ylang and neroli can help you unwind. Headaches due to nervous tension are also helped by these oils, but keep in mind that headaches can result from many causes, from indigestion to hormonal problems, and should be treated appropriately.

Relaxing/Antidepressant Formula

3 drops lavender
3 drops neroli
2 drops marjoram
2 drops ylang-ylang
1 drop chamomile
2 drop clary sage
1 ounce carrier oil

This can be used as a massage or bath oil.

Neuralgia, or nerve pain, is best remedied by treating the cause, although essential oils do alleviate the pain, especially when used in conjunction with massage.

Neuralgia Relief

5 drops helichrysum
3 drops chamomile
2 drops marjoram
2 drops lavender
1 ounce carrier oil

Combine ingredients and use for massage.

Herbal Adjuncts—Herbs can stimulate or relax the nervous system. A number of plants are relaxing, including California poppy (completely safe, with no addictive alkaloids), hops, valerian, passionflower and catnip.

One of the best tonics to repair the nervous system is wild oats (even eating oatmeal does some good); others include skullcap and vervain. St. John's wort repairs damaged nerves and helps overcome depression.

Glandular System

In his book *The Holistic Herbal*, David Hoffmann states: "It is in the complexities of our inner control systems that mind meets body most closely. If consciousness is seen as a faculty of the brain, then the partnership of nervous system and endocrine glands acts as a bridge linking consciousness and body." The glandular system includes the pituitary, thyroid, parathyroid, adrenals, pancreas, pineal, thymus and gonads (ovaries or testes). Endocrine glands secrete and release hormones directly into the bloodstream. Receptor sites for different hormones in each cell trigger changes or reactions in the cell's metabolism. Fatigue is probably the biggest complaint of North Americans and often results from overworked adrenals. Jobs, family, noise pollution and the stresses of today's busy lifestyles all contribute. Drinking coffee and other caffeine beverages puts an extra burden on already overworked adrenal glands.

Pine and spruce help revive adrenals. A massage or bath with the blend given below supports adrenal function—but don't forget to schedule time to relax!

Adrenal Support

4 drops pine (*Pinus sylvestris*)
4 drops spruce (*Picea mariana*)
2 drops lavender
1 ounce carrier oil

This blend can be used in the bath or as a massage. For extra stimulation, add 2 drops rosemary.

Herbal Adjuncts—Regulating the thyroid with essential oils alone may not be enough. Use an eclectic approach of herbs, diet and exercise for best results. For underactivity, some aromatherapists use seaweed absolute diluted to 3 percent and applied to the thyroid, although eating seaweed itself is more often recommended.

Digestive bitters—golden seal, dandelion and yellow dock, for examples—are useful here, acting through reflex stimulation. Beneficial herbs for the adrenals include ginseng and licorice. Add garlic, onions and seaweeds such as kelp, dulse, hiziki and wakame to your diet to boost an underactive thyroid.

Urinary Tract

The urinary system, consisting of the kidneys and bladder, regulates the body's water content and salt balance, and eliminates waste. The kidney determines what will be eliminated and what will be recycled. It is also involved in regulating blood pressure.

Antiseptic diuretics to treat bladder infections include cedarwood, tea tree, bergamot and fennel. Unlike some urinary herbs used to treat infection, such as uva ursi, these essential oils work well in both an acid and an alkaline environment. This means that they can be used in conjunction with cranberries, which acidify the urine. Use these oils preventively in a regular bath or a sitz bath.

Bladder Infection Relief

6 drops tea tree
2 drops thyme linalol
2 drops juniper
2 drops clove
2 drops oregano
1 ounce carrier oil (calendula is one of the best choices)

Mix the oils. Use as a massage oil over the bladder area twice per day. However, get professional help if there is a chance that you have a kidney infection.

Herbal Adjuncts—Use essential oils as part of a more comprehensive healing program that includes herbs and diet. The use of soothing herbal teas is a welcome adjunct to any treatment. Examples are plantain, marshmallow root and corn silk (yes, the hairy stuff under the husk; eat it fresh—it tastes just like corn—or make it into tea).

"Kidney stones" are mineral deposits most often composed of crystallized calcium and uric acid (or the amino acid cystine). Diet seems to be the primary cause, but excess weight, an inherited tendency and previous kidney infections are all potential contributing factors. Studies in Paraguay, where rosemary is an important folk medicine, found that this herb inhibits 95 percent of urease (found in alkaline and infected urine), and probably the formation of some urinary stones. Lemon and grapefruit help reduce the size of kidney stones and help prevent infection.

To treat a bladder infection, use uva ursi, yarrow, and goldenrod flowers. A good urinary tract tonic is a tincture or tea of dandelion, nettle leaf, fresh oats and rose hips. Hydrangea root, stone root, wild yam, cramp bark, corn silk and plantain leaf help eliminate kidney stones, but this condition may require professional help.

Reproductive System

Among the most common problems for women are those involving the reproductive system. As women with personal experience in this area, we will focus first on several female problems. This topic has been the subject of many good books; we recommend *Herbal Healing for Women* by Rosemary Gladstar, *Herbal for the Child-Bearing Years* by Susun Wees and *Hygeia: a Woman's Herbal* by Jeannine Parvati Baker (see bibliography).

PMS and Menstrual Cramps

The more researchers learn about hormonal substances called *prostaglandins*, the more obvious it becomes that they can cause PMS (premenstrual syndrome) and menstrual cramps. Certain prostaglandins called PG2 can be responsible for headaches, bowel changes, nausea, breast tenderness, joint pain and water retention, and contribute to moodiness, irritability and alcohol cravings—all common PMS symptoms. Ginger, cinnamon, cloves, thyme and garlic lower PG2 and can be eaten in foods. Relieve menstrual cramps with essential oils of chamomile, lavender, marjoram and melissa. For depression associated with PMS, nothing is better than clary sage, but you may also try neroli, jasmine and ylang-ylang. If you experience water retention, use grapefruit, carrot seed and juniper. Any of these essential oils (except garlic) can be used as a massage or bath oil. If headache is among your PMS symptoms, try inhaling lavender, marjoram or melissa. (For best results with any PMS or menstruation remedy, begin using it a couple of days before symptoms are expected.)

For problems related to hormonal imbalance, treat the liver with carrot seed, rosemary, helichrysum and rose. To encourage menstruation, use clary sage. Most women's conditions benefit from the use of the balancing lavender, geranium and rose.

Menstrual Cramp Oil

4 drops lavender
2 drops marjoram
2 drops chamomile or clary sage*
3 drops geranium
1 drop ginger
1 ounce carrier oil (infused oil of yarrow)

Combine ingredients. Apply to abdomen, hips and lower back.

*See Materia Medica "Considerations."

Yeast Infections

Many women have experienced at least one bout of yeast infection, which is usually easy to control. Chamomile, lavender, bergamot and tea tree inhibited about 70 percent of candida growth in laboratory experiments. Although opinion varies among gynecologists as to whether common yeast infections can be transmitted between sex partners, it's safest to treat both individuals.

Douching has met with criticism in recent years because some gynecologists fear it can upset the normal vaginal balance of a healthy woman or spread infection into the uterus. If done gently, however, douching is a good way to treat vaginal infection. Be sure to suspend the bag no higher than shoulder level so that the flow of water isn't too strong.

An appropriate essential-oil blend can also be applied to the abdomen or used in a bath. Another recommendation is to soak a tampon—or better, a small, soft natural sea sponge—in water containing essential oils. Use two sponges and alternate, sterilizing sponges between use by gently boiling or soaking in vinegar with a few drops of lavender oil. (Rinse well before using.)

Tea tree or lavender are very effective for vaginal yeast. We recommend caulophyllum or yarrow oil as a carrier oil.

Yeast Relief

1 drop thyme (chemotype linalol only)
1 drop chamomile
1 drop lavender
2 drops tea tree
2 drops bergamot
1 drop geranium
2 cups of warm yarrow tea

Combine ingredients. If you don't have the chemotype linalol, don't replace it with other thymes—they are too strong. For a simpler recipe, use 4 drops each lavender and tea tree oils. Douche two times a day. You can also mix the essential oils in 1/2 ounce of an infused oil of calendula or in caulophyllum. Insert one dropperful morning and night. A panty liner is recommended during the day.

Vaginal Bolus

Boluses (see "Guidelines" chapter) are effective treatments for a host of vaginal problems, especially cervical dysplasia (irregular cell growth on the cervix, which is precancerous). *Eucalyptus polybractea* (cryptone type) is one of the best remedies. This recipe can be customized to treat specific infections.

Bolus Recipe

2 teaspoons calendula blossoms
1 teaspoon goldenseal root
1 teaspoon yarrow leaves or flowers
8 drops tea tree oil
8 drops Eucalyptus polybractea (cryptone type)
1/4 cup cocoa butter

If this type of eucalyptus is not available, replace it with lavender or use 16 drops of tea tree.

Poor Circulation

Many female complaints are due to what Traditional Chinese Medicine (TCM) calls "blood stagnation." This basically means poor circulation in the abdomen, which contributes to problems such as hemorrhoids and pelvic inflammatory disease (PID). Use castor oil packs and sitz baths with essential oils (see below) to stimulate circulation. (For an understanding of TCM, we recommend Leslie Tierra's book *Herbs for Life*.)

Sitz Bath—A sitz bath can decrease menstrual cramps, PID and hemorrhoids. The bath requires two tubs large enough to sit in with water covering the abdomen. Fill one tub with hot water, the other with cold. Switch back and forth between the hot and cold tubs about four times. We find that four minutes in the hot and one minute in the cold is tolerable, and actually feels good after a few rounds. (You will soon want the hot hotter and the cold colder!) When you get out, your midsection will be bright red with blood circulation. When I (Mindy) had PID, this was the only thing that provided relief from the pain. This routine should be repeated as often as possible during the day.

Castor-Oil Pack—Getting results from using a castor-oil pack requires dedication and a little mess, and can take weeks or even months to produce results. Still, it can work wonders on pain from internal scar tissue, ovarian cysts, fibroids and even infection. You will need enough cotton flannel—several layers thick—to cover the abdomen, and about two cups of castor oil. Warm the oil, then dip the flannel to thoroughly soak it. Wring slightly to remove excess oil (it shouldn't drip). Place the flannel over the abdomen and cover with a piece of plastic, then a heating pad. Leave the pack on 30 minutes to one hour. When done, wrap the flannel in a plastic bag. After removing it from the bag, it may be reheated in a low oven. Replace every two weeks or so, depending on how much you reuse it. We like to use essential oils with castor oil packs. Add one-quarter teaspoon of essential oils to two cups of castor oil before making the pack. Lavender is a good choice.

Menopause

Menopause symptoms can include hot flashes, bone fragility, confusion, depression and a dry, less elastic vagina with a thinner lining—all caused by the erratic hormone activity. Both dry skin and vagina need a rejuvenating massage oil or cream. The hormone balancers geranium and lavender help menopausal symptoms. Pharmacologist Tony Balacs states that many essential oils have hormonelike activity, and speculates that their structure is so similar to the hormone's that they interact with the same receptors. Estrogenic oils include clary sage, sage, anise, fennel, angelica, coriander, cypress and niaouli (a type of tea tree oil).

Herbal Adjuncts—Beneficial uterine tonics include raspberry leaves, false unicorn root and motherwort. Herbs that help promote a normal menstrual flow are blue cohosh and partridge berry. Herbs that slow excessive menstrual flow or bleeding after birth include shepherd's purse and lady's mantle.

Good remedies for PMS or cramps are gamma-linoleic acid (GLA) (found in evening primrose, black currant and borage-seed oils), vitex, wild yam root, red raspberry leaf, licorice root and cramp bark.

Nine Essential Oils for Women's Complaints

Rose	universal female tonic and balancer, suitable for all gynecological problems
Clary sage	depression, PMS, menopause, postpartum blues (avoid long-term use if you have fibrocystic breasts or uterine fibroids)
Marjoram	antispasmodic, headache, menstrual cramps, constipation
Chamomile	anti-inflammatory, soothes frayed nerves, PMS, migraine
Lavender	overall equalizer, skin care, shock
Geranium	hormone balancer, menopause, PMS, yeast
Tea tree	antibacterial, herpes, the best yeast remedy, cystitis
Bergamot	widely antiseptic, water retention, yeast, depression
Neroli	insomnia, depression, anxiety, stretch marks

The best hormonal normalizer is vitex, suitable for almost any reproductive-system condition, and especially useful for treating PMS, irregular menstruation, cervical dysplasia, uterine fibroids and menopause. Herbs for balancing menopausal hormones are black cohosh, ginseng, dong quai, Siberian ginseng, licorice, fenugreek seed and hops. Vitamin E is also useful.

Pregnancy

Inhaling spearmint helps alleviate morning sickness; neroli and lavender can be very soothing throughout pregnancy and during labor. See "Massage" chapter for a recipe for massage oil for pregnant bellies. (See the "Guidelines for Use" chapter for contraindications in pregnancy and for information about which oils are safe to use.)

Herbal Adjuncts—In the first trimester of pregnancy, use gentle herb teas such as chamomile and lemon balm to deal with the usual maladies, but avoid strong emmenagogue (menstrual flow-inducing) herbs such as pennyroyal, rue, wormwood, goldenseal, juniper, sage and tansy. Recommended herbs for threatened miscarriage include black haw, cramp bark and false unicorn root. Toning and nutritive pregnancy herbs include raspberry, rose hip, chamomile, wild oat, nettles and partridge berry. For morning sickness, try an herbal tea of meadowsweet, spearmint, ginger and chamomile.

Lactation

Oils of anise, dill and fennel, used in a bath or massage, will ensure a healthy supply of milk for your baby. The herbs themselves can also be added to food or made into tea. Drinking herbal teas not only can increase the quality of your milk, but will also increase the fluids you need in your body to create it. Sage helps decrease lactation when you are ready to wean your baby. (Drink at least 2 cups of tea per day.)

Prostatitis

Prostatitis (inflammation of the prostate) can be helped by aromatherapy when combined with herbs and nutrition. An herbal sitz bath with chamomile and rosemary reduces inflammation, stimulates circulation and relaxes muscles in the pelvic region. Not quite as effective but more practical for some men is a warm compress or a massage oil applied behind the scrotum. Research has shown that muscle relaxation is vital in relieving a prostate that is chronically inflamed because of hormone imbalance. Be sure to have a doctor check this condition before attempting self-treatment.

Prostate Oil

5 drops lavender
3 drops pine
3 drops German chamomile
1 ounce calendula oil

Mix oils and apply to the area near the prostate twice daily to help reduce inflammation.

Male Hormonal Tonic

2 drops niaouli
5 drops pine
3 drops sandalwood
2 drops myrtle
1 drop patchouli (optional)
1 ounce carrier oil

Use daily in the bath or as a massage or body oil.

Herbal Adjuncts—For an inflamed prostate, drink a tea (or take a tincture or pills) of saw palmetto berries, nettle root, sarsaparilla root, uva ursi leaves and echinacea root.

Viral Skin Infections

Genital warts are caused by the human papilloma virus (HPV), and affect both men and women. They're difficult to detect at first, but turn white when dabbed with a half-vinegar, half-water mixture. Essential oils offer one of the most effective antiviral treatments for common or genital warts. Apply oils with a glass-rod applicator, dropper or a cotton-tipped swab two to four times daily—and apply only to the wart itself, as the oils can burn sensitive skin. Protect the surrounding area with salve. Have genital warts removed by a doctor if the oils don't eliminate them. They can be passed to sexual partners and can cause cervical dysplasia.

Genital-Wart Oil

5 drops thuja essential oil
10 drops tea tree essential oil
1/4 ounce castor or caulophyllum oil
800 IU vitamin E oil

Combine ingredients. The vitamin E facilitates healing and can be obtained by opening two 400-IU capsules.

Herpes

Herpes is a viral infection common among both men and women. *Herpes simplex* manifests around the mouth (cold sores) or the genitals. The painful *Herpes zoster* (shingles) is caused by the chicken-pox virus. Both strains can lie dormant in the nervous system and are often triggered by stress.

Herpes Formula

4 drops *Eucalyptus citriodora*
4 drops MQV (niaouli)
1 drop geranium
2 drops tea tree
2 drops bergamot
1 ounce carrier oil (calendula-infused oil is best)

Apply to affected area two or three times a day.

Miscellaneous Complaints

Cuts and Scrapes

A spray of diluted essential oils makes an excellent antiseptic. The germ-killing abilities of essential oils high in terpenes, such as tea tree, lavender, eucalyptus and lemon, increase when a 2-percent solution is sprayed through the air. The antiseptic quality of tea tree actually increase in the presence of blood and pus. Superficial cuts, scrapes and burns may also be treated with a salve. Although studies show that oils are antiseptic when diluted in an alcohol base instead of oil, this may sting in cases of an open wound. Tea tree, lavender, helichrysum, cistus, eucalyptus, rose geranium, sandalwood and rose repair skin damage and encourage new cell growth for faster healing.

Antiseptic Skin Spray

15 drops tea tree or eucalyptus
10 drops helichrysum
5 drops lavender
2 ounces distilled water
1/2 ounce grain alcohol or goldenseal tincture

Combine and shake well before each use to help disperse the oils. Spray as needed on minor cuts, burns and abrasions to prevent infection and speed healing.

Fungal Infections

Treat fungal infection with tea tree, lavender, eucalyptus, myrrh and geranium. Small amounts of peppermint relieve itching. Soak a compress in these essential oils diluted in vinegar, which also deters fungus, and apply to the affected area. A fungal powder is also appropriate to keep the area as dry as possible.

Antifungal Powder

1/4 cup bentonite clay
1 tablespoon goldenseal root powder
12 drops (1/8 teaspoon) each essential oils of:
- tea tree
- clove
- geranium

Combine all the ingredients and powder the affected area liberally. For fungal conditions, such as athlete's foot, an aromatic foot bath is a great treat.

Soak Those Pups

5 drops tea tree oil
5 drops sage
2 drops peppermint

Fill a portable basin or tub with hot water—or, better yet, sage tea. Add essential oils to water and soak for at least 15 minutes. For feet that sweat excessively, finish with a foot powder.

Rashes Caused by Poisonous Plants

The menthol in peppermint relieves the painful burning and itching of poison oak, ivy or sumac. A 2- to 3-percent dilution (12-24 drops per ounce) in vinegar or witch hazel provides blessed relief to nerve endings. Four cups of quick-cooking oats (they dissolve best) wrapped in a muslin cloth and/or one cup Epsom salts may also be added to a lukewarm bath, or mix a smaller amount and sponge on. Lavender and a few menthol crystals added to a tincture of jewelweed or sassafras are also helpful during the first stages of a reaction. Oil-based products aren't usually recommended, although some people find that a lotion relieves itching during the later, dry stage of poison oak, ivy and sumac.

Poison Oak/Ivy/Sumac Remedy

3 drops each:
- lavender
- helichrysum
- Roman chamomile
- geranium
- cypress
- 1/2 teaspoon salt
- 1 tablespoon water
- 1 tablespoon vinegar
- 1/2 teaspoon menthol crystals
- 1 ounce calendula tincture

Combine ingredients. Apply externally as needed. When healing begins, apply externally 6 drops each stoechas lavender and cistus (diluted to 2 percent) in aloe gel or juice.

Herbal Adjuncts—Take liver herbs such as milk thistle, burdock and dandelion; avoid sweets and fruits. Take vitamin C and pantothenic acid.

Inflammation and Burns

For inflammation, immediately apply a cold herbal compress with an anti-inflammatory oil, such as chamomile, lavender or marjoram. The first step in treating burns and sunburns is to quickly immerse the area in cold water containing a few drops of one of these essential oils, or to apply a cold compress that has been soaked in that water. Lavender oil and aloe-vera juice promote new cell growth, reduce inflammation and stop infection. Aloe, which is so healing it has even been used successfully to treat radiation burns, also contains the natural "aspirin," salicylic acid.

Sunburn Spray

50 drops (1/2 teaspoon) lavender oil
4 ounces aloe-vera juice
1 teaspoon vitamin E oil
1 tablespoon vinegar

Combine ingredients. Store in a spritzer bottle, and shake well before using. Use as often as needed to reduce pain and speed healing. Keep the bottle in the refrigerator for extra cooling relief.

Insect Bites and Other Critter Attacks

For mosquito or other insect bites that don't require much attention, a simple dab of essential oil of lavender or tea tree provides relief. Chamomile and lavender essential oils reduce swelling, itching and inflammation, and together with tinctures of echinacea and plantain often prevent an allergic response. (If an allergic reaction does occur, take 1/2 teaspoon of echinacea tincture internally.)

First-Aid Remedy

3 drops each:
  lavender
  tea tree
  German chamomile
  helichrysum
  1 ounce calendula infused oil

Mix together. This remedy is excellent for skin irritation, bites, stings, burns, inflammation, bruises or scrapes.

Adding essential oil and tincture to clay keeps the medicine reconstituted, preserved and ready for an emergency. As the clay dries it pulls toxins from stings and bites to the skin's surface to keep them from spreading, while also pulling out pus or embedded splinters.

Clay Poultice

12 drops lavender essential oil
1 tablespoon bentonite clay
1 teaspoon each tincture of:
  echinacea root
  chamomile flowers
  plantain leaves

Put clay in the container to be stored. Add the tinctures slowly, stirring as the clay absorbs them. Add lavender oil, stirring to distribute it evenly. Store poultice in a container with a tight lid to slow dehydration; it will last at least several months. If the mixture does dry out, add distilled water to reconstitute it.

Nothing is more annoying than trying to enjoy the outdoors while shooing away pesky insects. Many people don't care for the smell of citronella, a traditional repellant, but this formula smells great.

Insect-Aside Bug Repellant

5 drops eucalyptus
2 drops orange
4 drops lavender
2 drops lemon
8 drops cedar
1 drop peppermint
1 drop clove
1 drop cinnamon
2 ounces carrier oil

Mix together and apply liberally. Keep out of eyes.

Few "creepy crawlies" can survive the following blend. Use for skin fungus, scabies or other nonspecific critters.

Cootie Oil

10 drops thyme linalol
3 drops lemon
5 drops lavender
5 drops rosemary
1 drop clove bud
1 drop cinnamon bark
2 ounces carrier oil

Combine ingredients. Apply as needed.

Herbal Adjuncts—Jewelweed leaves, garlic, black-walnut hulls and the lichen usnea are all specific against fungus, and can be used as an external wash or soak. For other herbal adjuncts, see the chapter on "Facial Care."

Ears and Eyes

Antiseptic essential oils such as lavender and tea tree can be diluted in olive oil and rubbed around the outside of—never in—the ear and over the lymph nodes on the side of the neck. If the ear problem is caused by a throat infection, be sure to also use an antiseptic gargle. Hot compresses soothe pain in the ears. Always treat both ears, even if only one hurts, and continue treatment for several days after the pain is gone to make sure the condition does not return.

Aromatherapy Ear Rub

3 drops lavender
3 drops tea tree
6 drops Roman chamomile
1 ounce carrier oil

Rub around the ear and down the side of the neck. Apply one drop to a piece of cotton and place in the ear after application of the Herbal Ear Oil (below). For children use half this dilution (6 drops total of essential oil in 1 ounce carrier).

Garlic is antibacterial, eases the pain and inflammation of a simple ear infection, and is the remedy of choice for the fungal infection called "swimmer's ear," a condition that typically creates lots of itching.

Herbal Ear Oil

1/2 ounce each:
garlic-infused oil
calendula-infused oil
mullein blossom-infused oil

Use olive oil as the carrier for this infusion. Warm the oil before dropping it into the ear. Heat a spoon under hot water, dry it and drop the oil into the warm spoon; now draw the drops back into the dropper and place two drops in each ear.

For eye problems such as sties or inflammation, use a compress soaked in anti-inflammatory hydrosols such as lavender, chamomile or rose water, a popular eyewash in the Middle East. If hydrosols are not available, tea bags of chamomile or regular black tea provide a quick compress. Steep them in warm water for a few minutes, place a tea bag over each eye and cover with a cloth.

Boosting Immunity

Natural remedies increase the body's resistance to disease by improving its ability to fight infection. No single essential oil will heal a person, but many plants have immune-modulating properties. As with any natural healing modality, essential oils should not be solely relied upon in cases of serious illnesses—but they may be integrated into any therapeutic program.

Lavender, lemon, bergamot, thyme, chamomile, pine, sandalwood, myrrh and vetiver stimulate production of infection-fighting white corpuscles. The antiviral action of certain essential oils is one of their most valuable attributes—especially since allopathic medicine has little to offer. Essential oils with terpenoid compounds are very specific, notably the citruses and pine oils, as well as some oils in the phenol group. (See the "Chemistry" chapter.)

Building health is the best insurance against contracting illness. The following blend helps build the body's natural resistance.

Basic Immune Tonic Blend

3 drops lavender
3 drops tea tree
2 drops bergamot
2 drops ravensare
2 drops eucalyptus
10 drops *Caulophyllum inophyllum*
1 ounce carrier oil (calendula-infused)

Use as a body oil daily in the bath as part of a health-maintenance program, or to treat acute conditions such as cold or flu.

Herbal Adjuncts—"Adaptogens" are defined as safe, beneficial herbs that have a balancing and toning action. There is some controversy over which herbs fit the criteria, but there is little argument against the *Panax* ginsengs (Korean and American) or Siberian ginseng. The immune tonics echinacea, myrrh, calendula, garlic, wild indigo, astragalus, shiitake and reishi mushrooms, schizandra berries and ligusticum all build resistance.

Children

Care must be taken in treating children with essential oils, although there are any number of safe ones. Use one-third to one-half the adult dose, or a 1-percent dilution (five or six drops of essential oil per ounce of carrier oil), and don't forget that citruses may irritate the skin. See "Guidelines" chapter.

Chamomile, melissa and fennel used as massage oil, or taken as herb tea, soothe a variety of tummyaches—and the problems that can lead to stomachaches, such as frayed nerves, anxiety and overexcitability. Colic, gas pains, nausea and food allergies are also good candidates for these remedies. A study from Israel found that a chamomile, fennel and melissa herb tea with licorice helps stop crying and fussing in infants with colic. Researchers think that essential oils relieve muscle spasms caused when babies swallow air as they eat. Nineteenth-century parents gave colicky babies a "gripe water" of dill, fennel or anise, and East Indian and Lebanese mothers still use dill to ease colic. A European carminative water contains fennel, chamomile, caraway, coriander and bitter orange peel, all known to kill bacteria and relieve flatulence.

Most digestive woes are helped by a simple tummy massage.

Tummy-Rub Oil

2 drops Roman chamomile
1 drop fennel
2 drops dill
1 drop melissa
1 ounce carrier oil

Mix together and massage the tummy gently.

A relaxing treatment for children before bedtime is a warm lavender and chamomile essential-oil bath. Most children love taking aromatherapy baths, particularly if they have their own personal blends, and may want to get involved in choosing and blending scents. Popular fragrances include orange, grapefruit and tangerine—all antidepressants and relaxants. (See the Baths section of the "Aromatherapy Body Care" chapter for proper dilution guidelines for kids.) Nature's gentle relaxant teas such as melissa, lavender and chamomile can calm a nervous, overstimulated, cranky child, make headaches go away, or gently induce sleep—as well as help soothe a worn-out parent!

A child suffering from a headache, sleeplessness or overexertion will find relief in a cool compress of lavender placed on the forehead. Frankincense used in a vaporizer or as a massage oil is safe and effective for respiratory congestion or infection, even for infants. Other safe essential oils for children include mandarine, marjoram, neroli, jasmine and petitgrain. Treat a fever, measles, chicken pox or mumps with a tea of yarrow, catnip, peppermint and elder flower; ginger with a touch of lemon juice is also effective. The soreness of mumps is relieved by syrups and gargles made from teas of thyme, rosemary or sage. Antiviral oils of melissa and bergamot have proven effective against the mumps and chicken-pox viruses. (If you use melissa, be sure it is the real thing and not citronella or lemongrass; these don't have the same healing properties.) Use these essential oils in a steam or make a tea from the herbs.

For teething pain, give chamomile tea and rub the gums with a little diluted clove oil on your finger.

The following formula may be used for swollen tonsils, mumps and other lymphatic swelling in the neck area:

Neck Wrap

2 cups warm water
8 drops lavender essential oil

Mix the water with the essential oil. While the water is still warm, soak a soft cloth, preferably flannel, in the water and wring it out. Wrap the cloth around the neck. Cover with a towel to hold in the heat. Remove before it gets cold. Repeat as many times as you wish.

European children were once given "dilly pillows" filled with aromatic herbs such as lavender and dill to send them off to dreamland. The scent was also considered a digestive. Add chamomile and thyme to prevent nightmares.

Dilly Pillow

1 cup total:
- lavender flowers
- hops strobiles
- lemon-balm leaves
- chamomile flowers
- dill seeds

Fold a 5" x10" piece of cloth in half and sew up the edges, leaving just enough room to stuff the herbs inside. Combine the herbs in equal parts to make 1 cup. Stuff the herbs into the material, then finish sewing it up. Place beside or under the child's regular pillow.

6

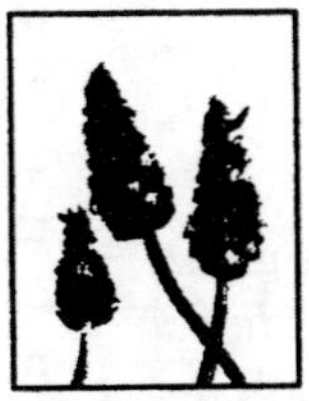

Aromatherapy Materia Medica

This chapter lists and describes the most important essential oils used in aromatherapy and thus summarizes the whole book. To help you, we've grouped together oils that are related either by genus or by association. The plant name appears alphabetically in a bold heading followed by the botanical name in italics. Historical or anecdotal information is followed by the individual headings described below. Other headings are also used where helpful (for example: "cosmetic/skin use," "associated oils").

FAMILY: This is the herb's botanical family. Some family names have changed, so we have indicated the previous name in parentheses to eliminate confusion.

EXTRACTION: The methods of extracting the essential oil and the parts of the plant used are listed. All of these methods are described in detail in the "Extraction" chapter. Finally, the fragrance is described.

MEDICINAL ACTION: The medicinal actions are summarized. Refer to the "Therapeutics" and "Guidelines" chapters for instructions on their uses and for sample recipes.

EMOTIONAL ATTRIBUTE: The commentary on the fragrance's emotional attributes comes from a combination of scientific study, historic folklore, personal experience and observations by other aromatherapists. This means that much of the commentary is unproved territory, but it is presented for your interest.

CONSIDERATIONS: These warnings are for the essential oil, but most of them do not apply to the herb itself, which may be substituted. Potentially toxic essential oils, which should be avoided altogether, are listed in the "Guidelines" chapter.

Angelica (*Angelica archangelica*)

Thought to have originated in Syria, angelica was one of the few aromatics exported to the Orient. The oil was a common flavoring and apothecary drug, and magical powers were attributed to it as the "root of the Holy Ghost." The way angelica hovers over the herb garden, it's no wonder! It offers little fragrance until you bite into a seed or snap a root. It still flavors Cointreau liqueur.

FAMILY: Apiaceae (Umbelliferae)

EXTRACTION: Distilled from root or seed. Absolute. The root oil is stronger and slightly more expensive, and it smells earthy/herbal; the seed oil is spicy/peppery.

MEDICINAL ACTION: Angelica regulates menstruation, is a digestive tonic and stops coughing.

EMOTIONAL ATTRIBUTE: The fragrance relieves depression (especially nerve-related) and provides a new outlook on problems.

CONSIDERATIONS: Use angelica very carefully: it can overstimulate the nervous system, and the root oil contains photosensitizing bergaptene.

Anise (*Pimpinella anisum*)

Originally from Asia Minor and Egypt, anise now grows throughout the Mediterranean. Turner's 1551 *Herbal* recommends it "maketh the breth sweter." The oil's delightful taste still flavors pharmaceuticals, confections, toothpaste, "licorice" candy in the United States, and numerous alcoholic beverages around the world such as French *anisette*, Turkish *raki*, Latin American *aguardiente*, Latvian *kummel*, Spanish *ojen* and Greek *ouzo*.

FAMILY: Apiaceae (Umbelliferae)

EXTRACTION: Distilled from the seed, anise has a sweet, licoricelike scent. The oil solidifies at room temperatures.

MEDICINAL ACTION: Anise is calming, and it reduces muscle spasms, indigestion and coughing. It is also mildly hormonal, increasing breast milk.

EMOTIONAL ATTRIBUTE: Smelling anise enhances relaxation, sleep patterns, emotional balance and even a sense of humor. It relieves stress from overwork. Said to be aphrodisiac, anise overcomes heartache.

CONSIDERATIONS: The oil can be narcotic and can slow circulation, so be careful. Although it may not be detrimental, it should be avoided by those with problems related to high estrogen. The anethole found in anise causes skin dermatitis in sensitive individuals.

Associated Oil:

Star Anise (*Illicium verum*)—This Oriental tree oil has similar chemistry and scent, so it sometimes replaces anise. It is distilled mostly from seed and occasionally from the star-shaped fruit. The related *I. religiosum* was once combined with rue and pyrethrum as a fumigant to keep bugs out of books.

Basil (*Ocimum basilicum*)

Basil comes from India, but has been cultivated in the Mediterranean for thousands of years and is now also grown in North Africa. The genus name *Ocimum* is probably from the Greek word "to smell." Once made into cleansing water for the hands and feet, it provides modern perfumes and soaps with an inexpensive substitute for mignonette (lily of the valley). The basils are so diverse in their scents, it has been suggested that they be classified according to chemistry instead of botany. You need to grow your own to have a complete collection, since only a few types are distilled. We have fun home-distilling a variety of spicy, citrus and fruity basils into hydrosols.

FAMILY: Lamiaceae (Labiatae)

EXTRACTION: Distilled from the leaf and flowering tops. The scent is sweet and spicy.

MEDICINAL ACTION: The scent relieves headaches, sinus congestion, head colds and resulting loss of smell. Basil treats herpes, shingles, nausea (even from chemotherapy), indigestion and sore muscles. Basil hormonally stimulates adrenals, menstruation, childbirth and production of breast milk.

COSMETIC/SKIN USE: Used for oily skin conditions.

EMOTIONAL ATTRIBUTE: Basil's uplifting effect overcomes a lack of confidence, indecisiveness, negative thoughts, stress, rattled nerves, hysteria and mental fatigue. It is said to increase awareness of one's surroundings. Gerard found the buoyant smell "good for the heart" and said it "taketh away sorrowfulness."

CONSIDERATIONS: Large dosages can be overstimulating and may eventually stupefy.

Associated Oils:

Reunion Basil (*O. basilicum*)—This variation from the Comoro and Réunion Islands (hence its name) has a harsher, more herbal scent. It flavors food and dental products. It contains very little linalol, but has 70-88 percent methyl chavicol, a skin irritant, so use carefully.

East Indian Basil (*O. gratissimum*)—Chemotypes of this East Indian species supply high percentages of thymol or eugenol.

Hairy Basil (*O. canum*)—From East Africa, this basil is delightfully spicy because of its high content of methyl cinnamate and camphor.

Bay (*Laurus nobilis*)

Also called "laurel," bay leaves were once placed on the heads of headache sufferers and Greek scholars. Today, we still confer a *baccalaureate* degree, which means "noble berry tree" in French. Crush a leaf and the smell is so intense it can produce a headache as easily as cure one. Apparently bay has even more interesting properties: the ancient Greek priestesses at Delphi sat over the burning fumes to increase their prophetic visions.

FAMILY: Lauraceae

EXTRACTION: Distilled from leaf (occasionally berry). Smells pungent and spicy.

MEDICINAL ACTION: Bay is a stimulant to lymph, sinuses, lungs, and circulation. It makes a very good liniment.

EMOTIONAL ATTRIBUTE: Smelling bay is stimulating and is said to improve memory.

Associated Oils:

Bay Rum Tree *(Pimenta racemosa)*—Also called "oil of pimento," this is the source of most commercial bay oil and the scent in Bay Rum cologne, which was originally from the Virgin Islands and made with rum. Cooler and sweeter than true bay, it scents bay soaps, cosmetics and colognes.

Allspice *(P. dioica)*—Familiar to cooks, this culinary seed tastes like a combination of cloves, cinnamon and pepper. It is the source of pimento water, an indigestion remedy in the West Indies and South America, where this evergreen grows. The name comes from the Spanish *pimiento* because the seed (actually a berry) looks like black pepper. It is sold as "Bay" oil.

Benzoin (*Styrax benzoin*)

The Arabs, who traded it for a frankincense substitute, called this Southeast Asia tree "incense of Java," or *luban jawi*. The Europeans interpreted this as *benjawi* and pronounced it "benjamin," then "benzoin." They made solid "vanilla" pomades from it. In India, the fragrance is sacred to the Brahma-Shiva-Vishnu triad, and Malays use it to deter devils during rice-harvesting ceremonies. The sweeter Sumatran *S. tonkinense*, especially the thick "almond tears," is considered better quality than the Sumatran *S. benzoin*.

FAMILY: Styracaceae

EXTRACTION: Solvent extracted from gum resin. Absolute, often thinned with ethyl glycol. It has a sweet, vanilla-like odor.

MEDICINAL ACTION: Once called "friar's balsam" because it soothes coughs and relieves lung congestion, a formula is still sold by this name. It is also used to treat poor circulation and muscular problems.

COSMETIC/SKIN USE: Benzoin is antiseptic, antifungal, protects chapped skin and increases skin elasticity.

EMOTIONAL ATTRIBUTE: This fragrance is for those who feel anxious, emotionally blocked, lonely or exhausted, especially from a life crisis. It creates a "safe space" that protects one from outside interference.

CONSIDERATIONS: Skin sensitizing.

Associated Oils:

Balsam of Tolu *(Myroxylon balsamum)*—A Colombian tree once cultivated by the Incas for its vanilla-like fragrance and medicine. The oil, distilled from the gum resin, treats lung congestion, scabies, eczema, and ringworm. Skin sensitizing.

Balsam of Peru *(M. balsamum var. Pereirae)*—This El Salvadoran tree got its name because it was shipped with Peruvian goods. The taste is hotter and more bitter than tolu. Skin sensitizing.

Styrax *(Liquidamber orientalis)*—The vanilla-like resin from this tree is used for indigestion, intestinal worms, poor appetite (especially due to illness), insomnia and menstrual irregularity. It can be toxic in quantity. *L. styraciflua* is the American variety. Skin sensitizing.

Bergamot (*Citrus bergamia*)

The small green fruit produced by this Mediterranean citrus tree aren't edible or pretty, but the smell they emit is wonderful! Unfortunately, you must live in a warm climate like California to grow them. First mentioned in the 17th century *En la Parfumerie Françoise*, the fruit was named after Bergamo, Italy, where the oil originated. It is still grown in Italy, mostly in Calabria.

Bergamot scents many colognes and flavors Earl Grey tea and some candies. Don't confuse this citrus with the common herb-garden bee balm *(Monarda didyma)*, also called bergamot.

FAMILY: Rutaceae

EXTRACTION: Cold-pressed from almost-ripe fruit rind. Fresh, clean scent.

MEDICINAL ACTION: An anti-inflammatory and antiseptic, bergamot enhances immunity; treats genital, urinary, mouth and throat infections, flu, herpes, shingles and chicken pox; and aids digestion. It is a traditional Italian folk medicine for fever and intestinal worms.

COSMETIC/SKIN USE: Bergapten-free bergamot is suitable on most skin conditions and eczema, and is a deodorizer.

EMOTIONAL ATTRIBUTE: Sniff bergamot to reduce depression, anxiety, insomnia or compulsive behavior cycles (including eating disorders). It balances emotions, instilling composure.

CONSIDERATIONS: Because it contains bergapten, bergamot is photosensitizing (i.e., may cause a reaction when skin is exposed to the sun). A bergapten-free essential oil is available.

Associated Oils: See Lemon, Orange and Orange Blossom.

Birch *(Betula lenta)*

This North American tree is the common source of Wintergreen oil, with which it shares similar chemistry, properties and fragrance. The formula for the popular 19th-century "Russian Leather" men's fragrance (so named because it kept book bindings soft) was closely guarded, but we now know it was mostly birch oil.

FAMILY: Betulaceae

EXTRACTION: Distilled from the inner bark after maceration in warm water. Sweet, sharp scent like some candies.

MEDICINAL ACTION: Birch is a muscular and arthritic pain reliever, a diuretic and a circulatory stimulant.

COSMETIC/SKIN USE: Birch is a skin softener that soothes irritation and psoriasis and helps prevent dandruff.

CONSIDERATIONS: Use this slightly toxic oil carefully and, because it smells like candy, be sure to store it safely away from children.

Associated Oils:

Birch Tar Oil—The thick tar is produced from the destructive distillation of bark, which involves burning and steam distillation, and produces a smoky odor. It is used on skin infections and infestations.

White Birch (*B. alba*)—This Northern European oil has different, less toxic, chemistry with similar properties.

Wintergreen (*Gaultheria procumbens*)—Native to northeastern North America, but a small and not very abundant tree, true wintergreen oil is rarely available and potentially toxic in large doses.

Calendula *(Calendula officinalis)*

The oil is costly and almost never available commercially, so we plant the colorful flowers in our gardens and infuse them into an herbal oil to use as a base for essential oils. Since two different flowers are called marigold, calendula is often confused with *Tagetes* (see Associated Oils, below), the oil of which is more common and also more toxic. Essential oil from both plants is often sold as "calendula."

FAMILY: Asteraceae (Compositae)

EXTRACTION: Absolute or CO_2 extraction from flowers. It has a pungent, fragrant odor.

MEDICINAL ACTION: Calendula relieves lymphatic congestion, inflammation and hemorrhoids, and is antiseptic.

COSMETIC/SKIN USE: Calendula heals skin wounds, rashes, inflammation and bites. Use it on oily complexions.

Associated Oil:

Marigold (*Tagetes minuta* and *T. patuh*)—This marigold is sometimes used on calluses, but the tagetone it contains makes the oil toxic and irritating, and the oil is phototoxic. Use calendula instead. *Tagetes* is high in beta-carotene (the precurser to vitamin A), is deep orange and sometimes sold as "carrot oil." It has recently become popular as an ingredient in perfumes. Use with caution.

Caraway (*Carum carvi*)

A medieval European love potion, facial water and cordial called Huile de Venus, this "oil of love" toned muscles and softened complexions. It was also sipped to quell indigestion. Today caraway seeds are more likely to find their way into rye bread than facial products.

FAMILY: Apiaceae (Umbelliferae)

EXTRACTION: Distilled from the seed, the fragrance is sharp and somewhat bitter.

MEDICINAL ACTION: Caraway relieves indigestion, colds, poor circulation, dizziness, some intestinal parasites, and nerve pain such as toothache.

COSMETIC/SKIN USE: A skin softener, caraway improves the complexion and decreases bruising.

EMOTIONAL ATTRIBUTE: The fragrance helps overcome mental strain and improves energy efficiency.

CONSIDERATIONS: Skin irritant.

Cardamom (*Elettaria cardamomum*)

Cardamom is a relative of ginger from the Middle and Far East, where it flavors Turkish coffee and East Indian chai tea. The seeds were a valued export item in ancient Greece.

FAMILY: Zingiberaceae

EXTRACTION: Distilled from the seed. Oleoresin. The best quality is sweet and spicy. Inferior seeds are more harsh, with a hint of eucalyptus odor.

MEDICINAL ACTION: Cardamom treats indigestion, poor appetite, diarrhea, coughs and muscular spasms.

EMOTIONAL ATTRIBUTE: An invigorating scent which East Indians have long considered an aphrodisiac.

Associated Oil: See Ginger.

Carrot Seed (*Daucus carota*)

Carrot-seed oil is distilled in France for use in perfumes. It comes from wild Queen Anne's lace, the ancestor of carrot. The carrot oil used in cosmetics is usually carrot root extracted into vegetable oil. Marigold (*Tagetes*) is sometimes sold as "carrot oil."

FAMILY: Apiaceae (Umbelliferae)

EXTRACTION: Distilled from the seed. The fragrance is fruity, sharp, pungent.

MEDICINAL ACTION: Carrot seed stimulates liver function, increases circulation and eases genital, urinary and digestive complaints. It is rich in beta-carotene, the precurser to vitamin A.

COSMETIC/SKIN USE: Carrot oil improves skin tone and elasticity, and moistens dry skin. It deters wrinkles, dermatitis, eczema, rashes and skin discoloration, and is used to treat precancerous skin conditions and ulcerated skin.

Caulophyllum Inophyllum

See the section on Carrier Oils in "Guidelines" chapter.

Cedarwood (*Cedrus species*)

This North American tree scents soap and cologne, although it has lost popularity since the 19th century, when even cedarwood "matches" were burned for their scent. The oil makes the wood resistant to wool moths and other insects.

FAMILY: Cupressaceae

EXTRACTION: Distilled from the wood. Resinoid, absolute. It has a soft, woodsy scent.

MEDICINAL ACTION: Antiseptic cedar treats respiratory and urinary infections.

COSMETIC/SKIN USE: Cedarwood is an astringent for oily and congested skin conditions, acne and dandruff. It relieves dermatitis, insect bites and itching.

EMOTIONAL ATTRIBUTE: Cedar increases emotional fortitude, self-respect and integrity, and stabilizes emotions by "grounding" an individual. It enhances meditative relaxation, intuitive work, and relieves stress, tension, aggression and emotional dependency.

CONSIDERATIONS: All cedars are best avoided during pregnancy.

Associated Oils:

Moroccan Cedar (*C. Libani*)—This is the legendary fragrant "cedar of Lebanon" once prized by Mesopotamians and other ancient cultures. The Phoenicians became rich controlling the forests and building ships for the Egyptians. After more than a thousand years of overharvesting, there are no longer enough trees to distill.

Atlas Cedar (*C. atlantica*)—This cedar oil comes from the Atlas Mountains in North Africa. With its pinelike scent closely resembling Moroccan cedarwood, it is considered the best cedar on the market.

Tibetan Cedarwood (*C. deodara*)—Also called "Himalayan cedarwood," Tibetan cedarwood has a warm, almost spicy fragrance and is the least toxic of all cedar oils. It is popular in India, where it grows wild.

Thuja (*Thuja occidentalis*)—Known as "cedar leaf" or "arbor vitae," this oil is distilled from leaves, twigs and bark. It contains the skin irritant thujene, which eliminates warts. It also contains thujone, a neurotoxic ketone, so it shouldn't be used by anyone prone to seizures. Thuja treats pelvic congestion, enlarged prostate, condyloma virus and urinary infections, but is potentially very toxic, so use with supervision or in tincture form. See also Juniper.

Celery (*Apium graveolens*)

Celery extensively flavors food, as well as alcoholic and soft drinks. It also scents soaps and some cosmetics.

FAMILY: Apiaceae (Umbelliferae)

EXTRACTION: Distilled from flower heads, celery's scent is warm, spicy and sweet. The absolute is blue-colored.

MEDICINAL ACTION: Celery is hormonal, stimulating lactation, and also helps relieve liver congestion, indigestion, genital and urinary problems, arthritis, rheumatism, gout and sciatic pain.

Chamomile, German (*Matricaria recutita*, formerly *M. chamomilla*)

German chamomile oil contains green-blue chamazulene (*azul* means blue), a potent anti-inflammatory constituent produced during distillation. In 1664, when chamomile was first distilled in glass, the distillers were surprised to see the blue color, which they previously thought was due to a reaction of the oil to the copper stills.

FAMILY: Asteraceae (Compositae)

EXTRACTION: Distilled from flowers. (The flowers are tiny, so they are usually accompanied by stems when distilled.) The odor is deep, sweet and herbaceous.

MEDICINAL ACTION: This versatile essential oil treats the inflammation of sore muscles, sprains, tendons and joints, as well as headaches, diarrhea, digestive tract ulcers, asthma and allergies. It helps reduce indigestion, PMS, menstrual pain, liver damage and children's hyperactivity. It also destroys various types of intestinal worms and improves immune system activity.

COSMETIC/SKIN USE: Chamomile is ideal on all complexion types, including sensitive, puffy or inflamed conditions. It also treats allergies, boils, rashes and enlarged capillaries.

EMOTIONAL ATTRIBUTE: This potent antidepressant helps those who experience oversensitivity, stress, anxiety, hysteria, insomnia or suppressed anger (especially when associated with the past).

Chamomile, Roman (*Chamaemelum nobile*, formerly *Anthemis nobilis*)—This short-growing perennial produces very little chamazulene, so the resulting oil is pale yellow, not blue. It is a digestive stimulant and antispasmodic used for constipation and insomnia. Its applelike fragrance gives chamomile the Spanish name *manzanita* ("little apple"). Medieval monks planted this species on the raised "healing beds" they made in their gardens for invalids to lie upon to relieve depression.

Associated Oils: The various types of chamomile are all antidepressants and anti-inflammatory; all treat burns, eczema and skin irritation.

Ormenis (*Chamaemelum mixtum*, formerly *Anthemis mixta* and sometimes *Ormenis mixta* or *O. multicaulis*)—Native to west Africa and Spain, ormenis is distilled in Morocco where it is also sold as "blue chamomile," although the oil is yellow, not blue. (The blue oil is probably *Tanacetum annuum*, also sold as blue chamomile.) There is some confusion about the genus and species of these oils, but hopefully importers will someday clarify their botanical origins. Less expensive than the first two chamomiles, both "blue" oils are anti-inflammatory. The related Tansy (*Tanacetum Vulgare*) oil is toxic and should not be used.

Artemisia Arborescens (*Artemisia arborescens*)—Commonly called "great mugwort," this oil is related to wormwood and mugwort. It has a sweet fragrance like the tanacetum annuum, and treats inflammation, bruising and pain. It contains potentially toxic ketones like those found in wormwood, so use it very carefully. A blue oil, it is also sometimes sold as "blue chamomile.".

Cinnamon (*Cinnamomum zeylanicum*)

In India and Europe, cinnamon was a popular aphrodisiac and antiseptic. Often fought over, it was the reason for the Portuguese seizing Ceylon in 1505, the Dutch later taking the country from them, and the British grabbing it next. Today, cinnamon is grown in Madagascar, Africa, Indochina and Sri Lanka. When this large, subtropical tree is two years old, it is harvested twice a year for 30 years. Small amounts of the oil spice up Oriental perfume blends. Eugenol isolated from the bark oil is turned into synthetic vanilla.

FAMILY: Lauraceae

EXTRACTION: Distilled from the leaf or bark, cinnamon has a sweet, spicy-hot fragrance. The hotter, more expensive bark is composed of 40-50 percent cinnamaldehyde and 4-10 percent eugenol. It is reddish-brown. The leaf is 3 percent cinnamaldehyde and 70-90 percent eugenol.

MEDICINAL ACTION: Cinnamon helps stop menstrual cramps, indigestion, diarrhea, and genital and urinary infections. It increases sweating, and creates heat when used in a liniment.

EMOTIONAL ATTRIBUTE: The smell relieves tension, steadies nerves and invigorates the senses. In very small amounts cinnamon can be an aphrodisiac.

CONSIDERATIONS: Both bark and leaf oils can irritate mucous membranes, but the bark oil is more hazardous. Use sparingly. Dermal irritant.

Associated Oils:

Cassia (*C. cassia*)—This less expensive cinnamon substitute comes from China as *kuei pi*, where it is medicine, seasoning and incense. It flavors cola drinks and lemonade, and scents Yardley's famous "Brown's Windsor Soaps."

Ceylon Cinnamon (*C. verum*)—From Ceylon, this antibacterial oil flavors mouthwashes, foods and drinks. Caution: it can be a skin irritant.

Camphor (*C. camphora*)—Unlike harsh mothballs (which are synthetic), the leaves and bark of "true" camphor are pleasant: woodsy with a hint of cardamom. The "fragrant" camphor from Formosa is even more pleasant, closely resembling rosewood. Long popular in China, where statues of Buddha were carved from camphor wood, camphor hydrosols in wine were digestive tonics, and chicken is still flavored by steaming it over camphor leaves. We've distilled the leaves of "fragrant" camphor into hydrosols for room fresheners and facial astringents. The Chinese harvest it by topping instead of felling the trees, although demand declined with the introduction of synthetic camphor in 1949. The odor counters shock and depression, and focuses one's attention. Arabs say it reduces sexual desire. Camphor is excellent for lymphatic massage, but it is also a heart stimulant, so use cautiously. White camphor can be used safely in small amounts, but don't use the more toxic brown or yellow camphor produced from heavier parts of the oil.

Borneo (Borneol) Camphor (*Dryobalanops aromatica*)—Used against plague and serious digestive infections, Marco Polo called borneo camphor the "balsam of disease." The Chinese burn the incense during funerals and important ceremonies. They also use it to treat wounds, sprains, infectious disease and nerve pain, as well as nervous exhaustion. It is distilled from an exudation of the mature trees. Younger trees produce a pale-yellow liquid camphor, not readily available.

Clary Sage (*Salvia sclarea*)

Clary sage was mixed with ambergris, cinnamon, brandy and sugar into a popular European cordial for digestive problems and to improve the complexion. It still flavors muscatel wine and tobacco; the largest U.S. grower is the tobacco company R. J. Reynolds. Another sage is also called "clary," but true clary oil comes from the thick-leafed herb, not this more delicate, tricolored leaf imitator.

FAMILY: Lamiaceae (Labiatae)

EXTRACTION: Distilled from flowering tops and leaves. Similar to ambergris, the winelike scent is sweet and heady. Concrete, absolute.

MEDICINAL ACTION: Clary eases muscle and nervous tension, pain, menstrual cramps, PMS and menopause problems such as hot flashes. It also stimulates adrenals and is a European remedy for sore throat.

COSMETIC/SKIN USE: Use the oil for mature or acne complexions, inflammation and dandruff. It rejuvenates cells and is also said to encourage hair growth.

EMOTIONAL ATTRIBUTE: Panic, paranoia, mental fatigue, general debility, postpartum depression and PMS are a few of the stress-related conditions clary sage is used to treat. Clary produces relaxation, dramatic dreams, euphoria, smiles—we pass it around classes to perk up the students! (It improves communication, once the giggling dies down.) Small amounts relax children. Herbalist William Turner said that clary sage "comforts the vital senses, helps the memory [and] quickens the senses."

CONSIDERATIONS: Large amounts can actually stupefy a person. Combined with alcohol, clary can increase drunkenness and nightmares, and in lab studies, it potentiates hypnotic drugs. Because of its estrogenic action, those who suffer from breast cysts and uterine fibroids or other estrogen-related disorders should avoid long-term use.

Associated Oil: See Sage.

Clove Bud (*Syzygium aromaticum*, formerly *Eugenia caryophyllata*)

Clove was the tree that Pierre Poivre risked his life to steal from the Dutch colonies. Today's supply comes mostly from trees planted on islands off Africa by the British. Once established, the trees bear their woody buds for at least a century. To discourage Indonesians from chewing betel nuts, the Dutch introduced cigarettes spiced with cloves, which were even more harmful than tobacco by itself. A popular 16th-century Italian cologne combined clove with lavender, musk and ambergris. The 19th-century "Guard's Bouquet" was a similar formula, dabbed on handkerchiefs. Simply inhaling the fragrance was once said to improve eyesight and keep away the plague—European doctors wore leather beaks filled with cloves and other aromatics to stave off infection. Envoys to the Chinese Han court held cloves in their mouths during audiences with the emperor to sweeten their breath. Europeans, East Indians and Chinese still freshen their breath and eliminate toothache with clove. Its constituent, eugenol, kills germs and pain.

FAMILY: Myrtaceae

EXTRACTION: Distilled from the immature flower bud, or steam distilled from the leaf or stem. The scent is powerful, spicy and hot. Concrete, absolute, oleoresin comes from buds. The leaf is highest in eugenol.

MEDICINAL ACTION: Clove relieves toothaches, flu, sore muscles, arthritis, colds and bronchial congestion. It destroys intestinal parasites and is a good addition to a heating liniment.

COSMETIC/SKIN USE: An antiseptic and antifungal, diluted clove oil may be dabbed on scabies or athlete's foot.

EMOTIONAL ATTRIBUTE: Small doses are stimulating, helping to overcome nervousness, mental fatigue or poor memory.

CONSIDERATIONS: The oil is irritating to skin and mucous membranes, so use it in 1-percent dilution or less.

Associated Oil:

Clove Bark *(Dicypellium caryophyllatum)*—A small Amazon tree called Brazil clove, sometimes used as a clove substitute.

Coriander (*Coriandrum sativum*)

Regardless of its reputation as a love potion, the 14th-century nuns of St. Just included coriander in their Carmelite water, a scent and complexion product that remained popular for the next four centuries. Coriander dominated Eau de Carnes cologne, a longtime Paris favorite, and still is used in the modern Coriandré perfume. It may seem a surprising choice for a fragrance, let alone an aphrodisiac, but the secret is to blend it with other oils. Grown in Russia, coriander is used mostly as a flavoring and to provide the materials to manufacture many synthetic fragrances. It scents soaps and deodorants.

FAMILY: Apiaceae (Umbelliferae)

EXTRACTION: Distilled from the seed. It has a distinct spicy, sharp odor.

MEDICINAL ACTION: Coriander soothes inflammation, rheumatic pain, headaches, cystitis, flu, urinary inflammation, intestinal gas and diarrhea, and is antiseptic.

EMOTIONAL ATTRIBUTE: Uplifting and motivating, the scent relieves stress.

Associated Oil:

Cilantro—This oil is distilled from coriander leaves, the popular herb that flavors Mexican, Chinese and Thai foods.

Cumin (*Cuminum cyminun*)

Some perfumes use small amounts of cumin, which is native to Egypt and the Mediterranean. The seed is commonly used in Mexican and East Indian foods, and is traditionally used in the ancient Ayurvedic medicine of East India.

FAMILY: Apiaceae (Umbelliferae)

EXTRACTION: Distilled from the seed. The odor is biting, warm, spicy and green.

MEDICINAL ACTION: Cumin relieves indigestion and related headaches, liver complaints, obesity, poor circulation and fluid accumulation. It is slightly sedative.

EMOTIONAL ATTRIBUTE: The fragrance counteracts emotional and physical exhaustion.

CONSIDERATIONS: Use cumin carefully, because it can irritate skin and is slightly photosensitizing.

Cypress (*Cupressus sempervirens*)

The landscapes of southern France and Greece are graced with this statuesque evergreen. It has long been associated with death, and even today Egyptians use cypress for coffins, while French and Americans plant it in graveyards. Smoke from the burning gum was inhaled in southern Europe to relieve sinus congestion, and the Chinese chewed its small cones to reduce gum inflammation. Related to juniper, it is commonly found in men's cologne and aftershave lotions.

FAMILY: Cupressaceae

EXTRACTION: Distilled from needles, twigs and, sometimes, cones. Concrete, absolute. Its odor is sharp, pungent, pinelike and spicy.

MEDICINAL ACTION: Cypress treats low blood pressure, poor circulation, varicose veins and hemorrhoids. It alleviates laryngitis, spasmodic coughing, lung congestion, urinary problems and cellulite. It is antiseptic and deodorant, and reduces excessive fluids in the body associated with conditions such as diarrhea and runny nose.

COSMETIC/SKIN USE: Use cypress on oily skin or to reduce excessive sweating.

EMOTIONAL ATTRIBUTE: Cypress eases insomnia and grief, and increases emotional stamina, helping one to get on with life after an emotional crisis.

Eucalyptus (*Eucalyptus globulus*)

With more than 600 species, eucalyptus offers a variety of scents. The blue-gum variety is the most widely cultivated and produces most of the oil available today. It was introduced at the Paris Exposition in 1867 after the Melbourne, Australia, botanical garden's director suggested it as an antiseptic replacement for cajeput. He was right. The French government planted the trees in Algeria to ward off the "noxious gases" thought to be responsible for malaria. It worked, but mainly because the trees transformed the marsh into dry land, eliminating the mosquito's habitat. Australia's "blue forests" are named for the haze produced by the tree's essential oil, which mutes the surrounding scenery. Eucalyptus is used liberally in industrial preparations, aftershaves, colognes and mouthwashes.

FAMILY: Myrtaceae

EXTRACTION: Distilled from the leaf and small twig. The odor is pungent, sharp and somewhat camphorous.

MEDICINAL ACTION: A potent antiviral, antibacterial and decongestant agent, eucalyptus treats sinus and throat infection, fever, flu, chicken pox and herpes. Most liniments and vapor rubs contain it, or its component eucalyptol. It is specific for thin mucus with lack of thirst and chills.

COSMETIC/SKIN USE: Small amounts are appropriate for oily complexion and especially acne. It is an antiseptic on wounds, boils, insect bites and lice.

EMOTIONAL ATTRIBUTE: The scent increases energy, countering physical debility and emotional imbalance.

Associated Oils:

Eucalyptus Australiana *(E. australiana)*—Specific for lung congestion and sore throats.

Lemon Eucalyptus *(E. citriodora)*—The high percentage of citronellal gives this eucalyptus a wonderful lemony scent, making it an inoffensive bug repellant. It is also anti-inflammatory, antifungal and antibacterial, especially against *Streptococcus*. Unlike standard eucalyptus, the scent is relaxing. Lemon eucalyptus is the best choice when there are symptoms of heat, such as thirst, dryness, thick mucus and fever. It is also specific for herpes, cystitis and arthritis.

Dives or Broad-Leaved Peppermint *(E. dives)*—Of the two chemotypes, one is rich in cineol (also known as cuminol) and is specific for acne; the other is rich in piperitone, a toxic ketone. They look identical but have different scents.

Peppermint Eucalyptus *(E. piperita)*—Similar to dives, this one is used in mouthwashes and veterinary supplies.

Blue Mallee *(E. polybractea)*—The two chemotypes of this species are cuminol (also known as cineol) and cryptone. The cuminol type (sometimes known as "cineol type") is specific for sinus and bronchial congestion. The cryptone type treats genitourinary tract problems, including chlamydia and condyloma virus, cystitis, cervical dysplasia, and uterine and prostate infections. Some success has been reported in treating uterine fibroids.

Grey Peppermint *(E. radiata)*—Most commonly referred to by its Latin name, Eucalyptus radiata treats overall ear, nose, throat and upper-respiratory problems, acne, vaginitis, ear infections and herpes. Its action is cooling and anti-inflammatory.

Gully Gum *(E. smithii)*—An energizer and immune modulant, this species is very mild, making it a good choice for children or sensitive people. Useful in the treatment of muscle pain.

Fennel (*Foeniculum vulgare*)

A tall, feathery Mediterranean herb, fennel loves to grow by the sea. Italian fishermen brought it to California, where it flourishes along the coast. It is called "licorice plant" because of its taste and smell. A fennel water for digestion is still made in Europe.

FAMILY: Apiaceae (Umbelliferae)

EXTRACTION: Distilled from the seed. The odor is herbaceous, sweet and licorice-like. A bitter fennel oil is distilled from whole herb.

MEDICINAL ACTION: Fennel reduces obesity, water retention, urinary-tract problems, indigestion and babies' colic. Its hormonal properties (mostly estrogen-like) increase mother's milk and slightly stimulate the adrenals. It is used to inhibit appetite.

COSMETIC/SKIN USE: Fennel refines the complexion, especially of mature skin, and heals bruises.

EMOTIONAL ATTRIBUTE: Stimulating and revitalizing, fennel increases self-motivation and enlivens the personality.

CONSIDERATIONS: Since it can overexcite the nervous system and even cause convulsions, use fennel oil carefully. Individuals with nervous-system problems, epilepsy or estrogen-related disorders should avoid it.

Associated Oil:

Dill *(Anethum graveolens)*—Dill oil is distilled from the seed. This southwestern Asia/Mediterranean herb treats obesity, water retention and indigestion, and also refines the complexion. Early Americans chewed the seeds to inhibit appetite during church services. Babies with colic were given "gripe water"—a syrup of dill, fennel and baking soda—then put to bed on fragrant "dilly pillows" (see "Therapeutics" chapter) of dill, lavender and chamomile.

Fir (*Abies alba* and other species)

The balsam fir, better known as the "Christmas tree," is native to northern Europe. "Fir" essential oil is distilled from the twigs or needles of many different firs, and even from spruces, pines and other conifers.

FAMILY: Pinaceae

EXTRACTION: Distilled from needles. The odor is fresh, soft, forestlike.

MEDICINAL ACTION: Fir soothes muscle and rheumatism pain, increases poor circulation, inhibits bronchial, genital and urinary infections, and reduces asthma and coughing.

COSMETIC/SKIN USE: Sometimes used for skin infections.

EMOTIONAL ATTRIBUTE: Fir combines the senses of being grounded and elevated. It increases intuition, and releases energy and emotional blocks.

Associated Oils:

Canadian Balsam (*A. balsamea*)—The oil, distilled from the oleoresin, is sweet and balsamy with a distinct Christmas-tree smell, making it one of the favorites of all firs. The tree grows and is distilled in North America.

Siberian Fir (*A. siberica*)—This carries an especially invigorating fir scent.

Hemlock (*Tsuga canadensis*)—Often sold as fir, the hemlock tree is sometimes confused with the poison hemlock (*Conium maculatum*), which Socrates was compelled to drink.

Pine (*Pinus* species)—Pine, especially Scotch pine (*P. sylvestris*), is used in cleaning solutions, European bath preparations (it increases circulation) and liniments. Apathy and anxiety are replaced by peacefulness and invigoration when pine's sharp fragrance is sniffed. According to Dr. Daniel Penoel, pine—especially *P. sylvestris*—is used to treat male impotency.

Black Spruce (*Picea mariana*)—The stimulating, fresh scent treats muscle spasms, adrenal insufficiency and fatigue.

Terebinth (*P. palustris*, etc.)—This is turpentine, or resin from pine sap. For medicinal use, a much higher grade than paint thinner is used to treat body parasites and infections, and as a disinfectant. It is sometimes called "pitch pine."

Frankincense (*Boswellia carterii*)

An important incense since ancient times. It is also known as *olibanum* or "oil of Lebanon" (*oleum libanum*). This small tree grows on rocky hillsides in Yemen and Oman, although the finest quality still comes from North Africa, with some produced in Somalia.

FAMILY: Berseraceae

EXTRACTION: Distilled from oleo gum resin that hardens into "tears." Absolute, CO_2. The odor is balsamic, "soft."

MEDICINAL ACTION: Frankincense is antiseptic and anti-inflammatory to lung, genital and urinary complaints, digestive tract ulcers and chronic diarrhea. It is also used in the treatment of breast cysts and to increase menstruation.

COSMETIC/SKIN USE: Frankincense is excellent on mature skin and acne, and helps counter bacterial and fungal skin infections, boils, hard-to-heal wounds and scars, and distended varicose veins.

EMOTIONAL ATTRIBUTE: Used throughout the ages to enhance spirituality, mental perception, meditation, prayer and consciousness, frankincense fortifies and soothes the spirit as it slows and deepens breathing. It is said to release past links and subconscious stress.

Associated Oils:

OLIBANUM (*B. papyrifera*). This is the historical species from Punt..

ELEMI (*Canarium luzonicum*). This tropical Philippine tree is distantly related to frankincense and was used in ancient trade. The oil, distilled from the gum, now scents soaps and cosmetics, and sometimes flavors food. Resinoid, absolute. It treats congested lungs, inflammation, infection and mature complexions. Emotionally, it reduces stress and nervousness.

Galbanum (*Ferula galbaniflua*)

Resembling a giant fennel plant, galbanum was used in the ancient world as incense. Native to the Middle East and West Asia, it is cultivated today in Iran, Turkey, Lebanon and Afghanistan. It was used in pharmaceuticals, but now it is mostly known as a food flavoring and a perfume fixative.

FAMILY: Apiaceae (Umbelliferae)

EXTRACTION: Distilled from oleoresin, collected by incising the stem base. Persian oil is solid; the Levant type is liquid. Galbanum has a green, woody, spicy odor.

MEDICINAL ACTION: Galbanum soothes aches in the hands, feet, muscles and joints. It treats indigestion, respiratory disorders, asthma and poor circulation.

COSMETIC/SKIN USE: Promotes cell regeneration, and tones mature or irritated skin. It was once used to dress inflamed and abscessed wounds.

EMOTIONAL ATTRIBUTE: Galbanum relieves emotional tension.

Associated Oils:

Galbanol—This type of *Ferula galbaniflua* has had most of the terpenes removed, making it more water-soluble.

***Asafetida** (F. asafoetida)*—This East Indian herb substitutes for garlic in cooking and sometimes in medicine. Its name is from the word "fetid," and yes, it really does stink. Therefore, it is seldom used in aromatherapy, even though it is highly antiseptic.

***Zalou Root** (F. hermonic)*—This is considered an aphrodisiac in Beirut.

***Musk Root** (F. sumbal* and *F. gummose)*—This species is from the Caucasus region of southeastern Europe.

***Silhion** (F. species)*—One of the most valuable trade commodities in ancient Greece. Before it became extinct from overharvesting, this herb was used as a contraceptive.

Geranium (*Pelargonium graveolens*)

Seventeenth-century Europeans took a fancy to this tender African perennial, also known as "rose geranium," and propagated it in their greenhouses. The resulting hybridization increased the species to more than 600, which includes many rose types—the only ones distilled commercially. The oil varies, depending on growing conditions and species. The French planted it in Algeria and Réunion (or "Bourbon"), giving geranium from this area the name "Bourbon." It is also grown in Morocco and China. The Chinese oil is slightly less sweet but produces a good yield, making it less expensive. The pharmaceutical industry widely uses the component geraniol. This and other parts of the oil are sometimes used as an ingredient to make synthetic rose. Although the leaves of rose geranium resemble common geranium (hence its name), the two are only distantly related.

FAMILY: Geraniaceae

EXTRACTION: Distilled from leaves. Absolute, concrete. It smells like a rose-citrus-herb combination.

MEDICINAL ACTION: A light adrenal stimulant and hormonal normalizer, geranium treats PMS, menopause, fluid retention, breast engorgement and sterility. Just sniffing it may help regulate blood pressure.

COSMETIC/SKIN USE: A popular skin treatment, geranium reduces inflammation and infection of wounds, eczema, acne and burns, and it is used in the treatment of bleeding, scarring, stretch marks, fungus, lice, shingles and herpes. It balances all complexion types and is said to delay wrinkling.

EMOTIONAL ATTRIBUTE: The fragrance relieves anxiety, depression, discontent, irrational behavior and stress. More esoterically, it is said to balance a passive-aggressive nature, heal poor relationships and enhance one's perception of time and space. Often described as a sedative, some aromatherapists consider it stimulating or even insomnia-inducing. Others describe it as "balancing." The key to such discrepancies is usually dosage.

Associated Oil:

***Zdravets** (Geranium macrorhizum)*—"True geranium" is used in perfume and Bulgarian herbal medicine. Studies show it strongly inhibits *Staphylococcus, E. coli* and *Candida* infections. Antidiabetic.

Ginger (*Zingiber officinale*)

Native to the tropics, ginger's thin, broad leaves are attached to a surprisingly succulent, spicy rhizome. The herb originated near the Indian Ocean, but it is now grown throughout the tropics.

FAMILY: Zingiberaceae

EXTRACTION: Distilled from unpeeled, ground rhizome. Absolute, concrete and CO_2. The fragrance is spicy, warm and sharp.

MEDICINAL ACTION: Ginger oil treats colds, fevers, appetite loss, indigestion, nausea, and genital, urinary and lung infections, and is anti-inflammatory. It makes a warming liniment. It destroys many types of intestinal parasites. Studies show it increases drug and herb absorption, normalizes blood pressure and helps protect the liver.

EMOTIONAL ATTRIBUTE: Ginger is a stimulant and aphrodisiac.

Associated Oil:

Galanga *(Alpina officinalis)*—This native of China has actions similar to ginger. It is often confused with "false-ginger" *(Kaemferia galanga)* oil.

Helichrysum (*Helichrysum angustifolium*)

This flower, sometimes called "everlast" or "immortelle," is native to the Mediterranean and North Africa and is cultivated in Spain, Italy and Yugoslavia. A related species, *H. orientale,* is also grown for oil, while *H. stoechas* is sold as an absolute.

FAMILY: Asteraceae (Compositae)

EXTRACTION: Distilled from flowers. The French *H. stoechas* oil has an orange hue. Absolute and concrete are both brown-red. The pleasant fragrance is spicy, sweet, almost fruity.

MEDICINAL ACTION: Helichrysum treats infection and inflammation of chronic cough, bronchitis, fever, muscle pain, arthritis, phlebitis and liver problems, and counters allergic reactions such as asthma.

COSMETIC/SKIN USE: Helichrysum stimulates the production of new cells, so it is used on acne, scar tissue, bruises, couperose skin, mature skin and burns. It is used as a fixative in cosmetics and perfume. Extracts are added to sunscreens to protect skin from ultraviolet rays.

EMOTIONAL ATTRIBUTE: The scent helps lift one from depression, lethargy, nervous exhaustion and stress. Some aromatherapists say it helps drug detoxification, including nicotine.

Hyssop (*Hyssopus officinalis*)

Once considered sacred, this herb was often used in purification practices. Hyssop comes from the Mediterranean. Most of the oil produced goes into expensive perfumes.

FAMILY: Lamiaceae (Labiatae)

EXTRACTION: Distilled from flowering tops. The odor is spicy, strong, herbaceous.

EMOTIONAL ATTRIBUTE: A sedative, hyssop reduces grief and hysteria while increasing mental clarity.

CONSIDERATIONS: A nervous-system stimulant, use hyssop with caution: large doses may raise blood pressure and trigger asthma or epilepsy.

Associated Oil:

Hyssop *(H. officinalis* var. *decumbens)*—This variety of hyssop contains none of the hazardous ketones found in regular hyssop. High in linalol, it is a sinus and lung decongestant, safe for allergies, sinusitis, bronchitis, asthma and nervousness.

Inula, Sweet (*Inula graveolens*, or *I. odorata*)

This plant native to Asia and cultivated in many locales produces an essential oil that is strongly mucolytic. It is best dispensed from a diffuser for respiratory problems.

FAMILY: Asteraceae (Compositae)

EXTRACTION: Distilled from the root, resulting in a rich blue-green oil. The odor is strong and pungent, somewhat resembling eucalyptus.

MEDICINAL ACTION: Sweet inula relieves muscle tension, inflammation, sinus congestion, bronchitis, and high blood pressure. It is best used in the treatment of chronic, rather than acute, lung problems. A compound is used in Europe for the treatment of intestinal worms.

COSMETIC/SKIN USE: Relieves skin rashes, herpes and itching.

CONSIDERATIONS: High in potentially toxic ketones, so use only with supervision.

Associated Oil:

Inula *(I. helenium)*—This is the medicinal herb elecampane, commonly used for lung congestion. Because the essential oil was found to cause skin allergies in 23 out of 25 test subjects, we suggest using a tea or tincture of this herb instead.

Jasmine (*Jasminum officinale* and *J. grandiflorum*)

Probably an Iranian native, jasmine has captured the imagination for centuries. Forty-three different species are grown in East India, where women dress their hair with it and where it is poetically known as "moonlight of the grove." Also called the "king of fragrance," jasmine's complex scent is found in most great perfumes. The most prized oil comes from France and Italy, although about 80 percent is Egyptian. Try as chemists do to reproduce it, synthetic jasmine is so harsh that it demands a touch of the true oil to soften it.

FAMILY: Oleaceae

EXTRACTION: Enfleurage of blossoms. Concrete, absolute (separated from the concrete, then steam distilled). The fragrance is fruity, floral and sweetly exotic.

MEDICINAL ACTION: Jasmine is a nervous-system sedative that reduces menstrual cramps and is sometimes used to alleviate prostate problems. Culpeper suggested rubbing it into "hard, contracted limbs."

COSMETIC/SKIN USE: The absolute is used for dry, sensitive or mature skin.

EMOTIONAL ATTRIBUTE: Jasmine's fragrance soothes headaches, insomnia, depression, anger and worry, and dissolves apathy, indifference and lack of confidence. Also an aphrodisiac.

Associated Oil:

Chinese Jasmine (*J. sambac*)—Also called "sambac jasmine," this is originally from India and is richly fragrant.

Juniper (*Juniperus communis*)

The berries of this North American shrub flavor gin, named after *genièvre*, French for "juniper berry." Traditionally the fragrance was thought to ward off contagious diseases. Native Americans living in the high deserts of the West still burn it during purification and healing ceremonies. Until World War II, the French also burned it in their hospitals as an antiseptic.

FAMILY: Cupressaceae

EXTRACTION: Distilled from ripe berries. Resinoid, absolute. Its pungent, herbaceous, peppery odor is pinelike and camphorous. The berries offer the highest quality oil, but needles, branches and berries that have already been distilled to flavor gin are sometimes used.

MEDICINAL ACTION: Juniper is used in the treatment of arteriosclerosis, rheumatic pain, general debility, and congestion-related problems such as varicose veins, hemorrhoids, fluid retention and cellulite. It is a genital and urinary tract antiseptic, a circulatory stimulant, and it increases stomach acid.

COSMETIC/SKIN USE: Juniper is suitable for acne, eczema, and greasy hair or dandruff.

EMOTIONAL ATTRIBUTE: Juniper is good for those with mental fatigue, insomnia and anxiety and for those who are emotionally drained. It provides a feeling of protection when the demands of others pull too strongly.

CONSIDERATIONS: Juniper can be harsh on the kidneys, so choose a more gentle oil if they are inflamed.

Associated Oils:

Cedarwood, Virginia (*J. virginiana*)—This juniper is the real source of most "cedar oil"—and most wooden pencils! It scented the "Lebanon cedarwood" that perfumed many a Victorian handkerchief. A Texas cedarwood (*J. mexicana*) oil is also produced, while the low-priced East African *J. procera* scents soap and sometimes cologne. *J. sabina* is the most toxic of the junipers and should be avoided.

Oil of Cade (Juniper Tar)—Made by "destructive" distillation of the roots that involves burning the wood, the resulting thick, smoky tar was once used for infected wounds, eczema and skin parasites. Today, it provides foods with a smoked flavor.

Labdanum (*Cistus labdaniferus*)

Native to Spain and Greece, this is the "rockrose" grown in some North American gardens. Possibly the Bible's *onycha* and "rose of Sharon" (Song 2:1), it often replaces ambergris. It has long been popular in Spain, which remains the major producer today. Shepherds in ancient Crete would drive their herds through the plants so the sticky gum would collect on the animal's coats; after combing it out, they'd take the gum to market. Don't confuse this plant with laudanum, an old-time pain remedy made of opium.

FAMILY: Cistaceae

EXTRACTION: Leaves and twigs are boiled and the resin skimmed off, then aged to produce resinoid and absolute with a warm, spicy, balsamic odor. A fixative.

MEDICINAL ACTION: Labdanum is a nervous-system sedative, used in the treatment of rheumatism, colds, coughs, menstrual problems, cystitis and hemorrhoids.

COSMETIC/SKIN USE: Antiseptic to wounds, acne, dermatitis and boils.

EMOTIONAL ATTRIBUTE: Labdanum is both emotionally elevating and grounding. It improves meditation and intuition, and raises consciousness. It calms the nerves and promotes sleep, yet is also an aphrodisiac.

Associated Oils:

Cistus (*C. incanus*)—An essential oil with a lighter, more pungent odor distilled from the gum.

Cistus (*Helianthemum canadense*)—This oil, distilled from a plant called frostwort, is also called cistus. It is used for skin problems and precancerous skin conditions.

Lavender (*Lavandula angustifolia*, previously *L. vera* and *L. officinale*)

A well-loved Mediterranean herb, this English lavender has been associated with cleanliness ever since Romans added it to their washing water. In fact, the word comes from the Latin word *lavare* ("to wash") and is the root for the word "lavatory." Lavender remained a popular facial water from the 14th through the 19th centuries. The formula for the modern lavender water by Yardley adds attar of rose, musk and neroli. Today, Mitcham lavender of Surrey, England, produces an excellent quality oil. It is among the safest and most widely used oils in aromatherapy. When in doubt, use lavender!

FAMILY: Lamiaceae (Labiatae)

EXTRACTION: Distilled from flowers. Absolute, concrete. The odor is sweet floral and herbal, with balsamic undertones. The term "40-percent ester," often seen on lavender oil, means that it has a high ester content—boosted, if necessary, with natural esters that have been extracted from lavender.

MEDICINAL ACTION: Lavender treats lung, sinus and vaginal infections, including candida. It is an excellent treatment for laryngitis and asthma. It relieves muscle pain, headaches, insect bites, cystitis and other inflammation. It also treats digestive disturbances, including colic, and helps boost immunity.

COSMETIC/SKIN USE: Lavender is suitable for all skin types. A cell regenerator that prevents scarring and stretch marks, it has a reputation for slowing wrinkles. It is used on burns, sun-damaged skin, wounds, rashes and skin infections.

EMOTIONAL ATTRIBUTE: Nervousness, exhaustion, insomnia, irritability, depression and even manic depression are addressed by lavender. It is specific for central-nervous-system problems. For centuries, lavender was brought into the birthing room and made into baby pillows. Old texts say it "raises the spirit," and Victorian women revived themselves with lavender-filled "swooning pillows." William Turner suggested in his *Herbal* that lavender could "comfort the braine." A balancing oil, it both relaxes and stimulates.

Associated Oils:

Lavandin (*L. x intermedia* or *L. x hybrida*)—This is English lavender crossed with spike lavender. Such strains—such as Abrial, Super, Grosso (the most productive and common), Standard and Maime Epis Tête—have a slightly camphorous fragrance that is less refined than their parent lavenders. About 20 times more of the less-expensive lavandin is produced than true English lavender, which is more difficult to cultivate. Lavandin has similar, but less pronounced, healing properties; use it for muscle pain, and as a disinfectant and deodorant.

Spike Lavender (*L. latifolia*)—Sometimes called *aspic*, this camphorous species relieves congestion and is good for acne. It has a high yield, so is less expensive. It is grown mostly in Spain.

Stoechas Lavender (*L. stoechas*)—This oil is said to heal wounds and reduce inflammation, but is more toxic than other lavenders—so use cautiously.

Lemon (*Citrus limon*)

The lemon tree originated in Asia, but is now widely cultivated in Italy, Australia and California. The fragrance is popular in colognes and household cleaning products. The flowers have a pleasant aroma, but only the peel oil is produced commercially.

FAMILY: Rutaceae

EXTRACTION: Cold-pressed from fresh peel. The odor is distinctively sharp and citrus.

MEDICINAL ACTION: An antioxidant, preservative and antiseptic, lemon oil helps counter viral and bacterial infections. It treats hypertension with high blood pressure, congested lymph glands and liver, excessive stomach activity, and the immune system. It improves metabolism by reducing water retention, slowing weight gain and increasing mineral absorption.

COSMETIC/SKIN USE: Lemon is best used on oily complexions and for skin impurities. It treats bruises and skin infection.

EMOTIONAL ATTRIBUTE: The scent dissipates feelings of impurity or indecisiveness, and can stimulate emotional purging. It also increases one's sense of humor and general well-being. Like other citruses, it is antidepressive.

CONSIDERATIONS: Lemon can be photosensitizing and irritating to sensitive skin.

Associated Oil:

Cedro Oil—A terpeneless, more water-soluble lemon oil.

Lemongrass (*Cymbopogon citratus*)

Originally from India, lemongrass is an important medicine in South America and Southeast Asia. It is grown in Central America, Brazil and China, and is one of the ten best-selling essential oils in the world (about 1,500 tons per year). It is used in soaps, cosmetic fragrances and deodorants, and gives Ivory soap its familiar scent. The constituent citral is extracted from it.

FAMILY: Poaceae (Gramineae)

EXTRACTION: Distilled from partially dried leaves. It has a distinctive lemon-herbal, slightly bitter fragrance.

MEDICINAL ACTION: It is antiseptic and treats pain from indigestion, muscle cramps, rheumatism, nerve conditions and headaches. It is also an effective anticoagulant.

COSMETIC/SKIN USE: Lemongrass counters oily hair, acne, skin infections, scabies and ringworm. It is also deodorant.

CONSIDERATIONS: Nontoxic, but it causes skin sensitivity in some people. Lemongrass will burn the skin if not sufficiently diluted.

EMOTIONAL ATTRIBUTE: The fragrance is sedating and soothing.

Associated Oils:

Palmarosa (*C. martini*)—Palmarosa's lemon-rose fragrance is reminiscent of the richer, more expensive rose geranium, which it is often used to adulterate. The scent varies depending on its quality and age, and on whether it comes from India, Brazil, the Philippines or Java. Palmarosa treats stress and nervous exhaustion. A cell regenerator, it balances oil production and can be used on any complexion type, but especially for acne, infected skin or varicose veins. The constituent geraniol is extracted from it.

Lemongrass Cochin (*C. flexuosus*)—Grown in India primarily for isolation of citral.

Citronella (*C. nardus*)—While riding an elephant near the Egyptian border in 332 B.C., Alexander the Great supposedly became intoxicated when he smelled "spikenard." More likely, it was citronella being crushed underfoot. Known as "nard," citronella was first exhibited at London's Crystal Palace in 1851 and proceeded to become the primary scent in cleaning products. It is a physical and emotional purifier, used to treat colds, infections and oily complexions. Inexpensive citronella often adulterates lemon verbena and melissa, although it is distinctly camphorous and harsh, and can irritate skin. The preparation *Oleum Melissae Indicum* is actually made from citronella oil, not melissa.

Java Citronella (*C. winterianus*)—Widely cultivated because it yields twice the oil of the Ceylon type and is a little sweeter. A source of the constituent citronellal.

Lovage (*Levisticum officinale*)

This large European and west Asian plant is common in herb gardens. It tastes like a very strong celery. The herb is often used in treating women's complaints.

FAMILY: Apiaceae (Umbelliferae)

EXTRACTION: Distilled from fresh roots, or from leaves and stalks. The powerful fragrance is spicy, sweet, and reminiscent of angelica or celery.

MEDICINAL ACTION: Treats indigestion, digestive spasms and congestion, rheumatism, poor circulation and menstrual irregularity. Helps remove toxic accumulation and reduce water retention.

CONSIDERATIONS: Photosensitizing and potentially toxic. Use sparingly.

Marjoram
(*Origanum marjorana* or *Marjorana hortensis*)

"Sweet marjoram" is native to Asia but is a naturalized citizen of Europe, where singers preserve their voices with the honeyed tea. It was used in weddings to symbolize honor, happiness, and love. A marjoram species was probably the "hyssop" of the Bible, used for purification. It is an antioxidant food preserver.

FAMILY: Lamiaceae (Labiatae)

EXTRACTION: Distilled from leaves. Oleoresin. The odor is sweet, herby and a little warm, hinting of camphor.

MEDICINAL ACTION: A strong sedative, marjoram eases muscle spasms, tics, menstrual cramps, headaches (especially migraines) and stiff joints. Treats spasmodic coughs, colds, flu, laryngitis and hypertension, and is a light laxative. Also helps normalize blood pressure.

COSMETIC/SKIN USE: Use marjoram on bruises, burns and inflammations, and to treat fungal and bacterial infections.

EMOTIONAL ATTRIBUTE: Marjoram helps those who feel emotionally unstable or are prone to hysteria or irritability, especially due to outside stimulus. The old texts say it works so well that overuse deadens the emotions. Modern aromatherapists use marjoram to ease loneliness, rejection and a "broken heart."

Associated Oils:

Oregano *(O. vulgare)*—Closely related botanically, the division between the oreganos and marjorams is often hazy. However, true oregano is much more irritating to the skin. Although it is effective against respiratory, genital, urinary and intestinal infections, we suggest using less irritating oils.

Spanish Marjoram *(Thymus mastichina)*—Also called "wild marjoram," this North African thyme is antiseptic to upper-respiratory infection, but is not a sedative or muscle relaxant like sweet marjoram. It is also much harsher and less expensive. Several other species of thyme are also sold as "marjoram."

Spanish Oregano (*T. capitatus*). Called *origan* in the perfume trade, this is really a thyme with an oregano-like scent. It can irritate skin and should be used very cautiously, if at all.

Melissa (*Melissa officinalis*)

Well-known to herbalists as "lemon balm," melissa is a southern European native. A medieval favorite, it was the main ingredient in "Carmelite Water," along with lemon peel, nutmeg, coriander and angelica. It was used for nervous headaches and neuralgia, and to improve the complexion. It is still produced as *Eau de Mélisse de Carmes* and is found in *Klosterfrau Melissengeist* in Germany. Not easily distilled, the expensive, low-yielding oil is often adulterated with lemon or citronella.

FAMILY: Lamiaceae (Labiatae)

EXTRACTION: Distilled from leaves. The sweet smell is soft, lemony.

MEDICINAL ACTION: Melissa treats indigestion, lung congestion, high blood pressure, muscle spasms, menstrual problems, and sometimes infertility. It fights inflammation and viral infections such as strep, herpes and chicken pox.

EMOTIONAL ATTRIBUTE: Shock, distress, depression, nervousness and insomnia are helped by melissa's sedative action. Gerard (agreeing with Avicenna) said it "maketh the heart merry, joyful, strengtheneth the vitall spirits."

Associated Oil:

Lemon Verbena *(Aloysia triphylla,* formerly *Lippia citriodora)*—Similar in fragrance and cost to melissa, lemon verbena is often adulterated with less expensive oils. It is used on oily complexions and for nervous indigestion. The soothing fragrance encourages both sleep and concentration.

Mimosa (*Acacia decurrens var. dealbata*)

A common Australian tree—also called by the less poetic name "black wattle"—mimosa is grown in Africa, Europe and warmer sections of the United States. It is used mostly in perfume.

FAMILY: Mimosaceae

EXTRACTION: Absolute, concrete. The scent resembles straw or beeswax, with slightly bitter undertones.

EMOTIONAL ATTRIBUTE: Mimosa's scent is relaxing and helps overcome anxiety, oversensitivity, stress, and nervous tension.

Associated Oil:

Cassie *(A. farnesiana)*—This leguminous American plant is grown primarily in North Africa, and to a lesser degree in France. Also called "sweet acacia," it is similar to mimosa. Used in Oriental-style perfumes, it also treats depression, nervous exhaustion, stress and frigidity. Don't confuse cassie with the cassia related to cinnamon.

Myrrh (*Commiphora myrrha*)

This small, scrubby tree from the Middle East and northeast Africa isn't very handsome, but it makes up for its lackluster looks with the precious gum it exudes. An important trade item for more than a thousand years, myrrh was a primary ingredient in ancient cosmetics and incenses. The Egyptians mummified their dead with it.

MEDICINAL ACTION: Myrrh improves digestion, diarrhea and immunity. It treats coughs, gum disease, wounds, candida, overactive thyroid and scanty menstruation.

COSMETIC/SKIN USE: Myrrh is an expensive treatment for chapped, cracked or aged skin, eczema, bruises, infection, varicose veins and ringworm.

EMOTIONAL ATTRIBUTE: Myrrh has been used since antiquity to inspire prayer and meditation, and to fortify and revitalize the spirit.

Associated Oils:

Opopanax *(Illicium verum)*—This oil from Somalia and Ethiopia is sold as a low-grade myrrh. Lumps that exude from the root and stems are steam-distilled after hardening. Opopanax gives liquor a winelike taste and is a fixative. The herb that bears the name *Opopanax chironium* is a Sudanese and Arabian plant similar to parsnips, and isn't made into oil. To add to the confusion, cassie (*Acacia farnesiana*) is sometimes called "opopanax."

Copaiba Balsam (*Copaiba officinalis*)—This South American oleoresin (not really a balsam), called copal, is similar to myrrh. In Central and South America, where it has been used for centuries as incense, the Catholic church uses it in place of myrrh, and herb vendors sell it in almost every market.

Myrtle (*Myrtus communis*)

The Biblical Queen Esther changed her name to Hadassah, after the Hebrew word hadas, for "myrtle." This small, attractive North African tree now makes itself at home throughout the Mediterranean, and was a favorite in the ancient gardens of Baghdad, Granada and Damascus. Today, it is grown in Morocco. It was the main ingredient in the 16th-century complexion remedy called "Angel's Water."

FAMILY: Myrtaceae

EXTRACTION: Distilled from leaves, twigs and sometimes flowers. The scent is spicy and slightly camphorous.

MEDICINAL ACTION: Treats lung and respiratory infections, spasmodic coughs, muscle spasms and hemorrhoids.

COSMETIC/SKIN USE: Myrtle is appropriate for oily complexions, acne and enlarged surface veins.

EMOTIONAL ATTRIBUTE: The scent balances energy. The ancient Greeks and Romans honored poets with myrtle to suggest that their fame would never die.

Oakmoss (*Evernia prunastri*)

This lichen (a combination of a fungus and algae), which hangs from trees like Spanish moss, was found in Egyptian royal tombs. It is a fixative in chypre-type perfumes (named after Cyprus, the home of this moss) and was a popular 16th-century perfume. It is collected in Yugoslavia, France, Italy and Morocco.

FAMILY: Usneaceae

EXTRACTION: Absolute, concrete (vacuum-distilled from absolute). Offers an earthy, full and slightly sweet fragrance.

EMOTIONAL ATTRIBUTE: Creates sense of home, attachment, belonging.

Associated Oil:

Tree Moss (*E. furfuracea*)—This lichen has a sharper odor than oakmoss, especially when it grows on pines, which contributes a turpentine-like quality to the original bouquet.

Orange (*Citrus sinensis*)

The familiar sweet orange comes from Sicily, Israel, Spain and the United States, each offering a slightly different characteristic. *Chu-lu*, the first monograph describing the various citruses, was written in China in 1178.

EXTRACTION: Cold-pressed from peel. An inferior oil comes from peel pressed for juice. A more water-soluble, terpeneless oil is used in soft drinks. The scent is perky and lively.

COSMETIC/SKIN USE: Good for oily complexions.

MEDICINAL ACTION: Orange treats flu, colds, congested lymph, irregular heartbeat and high blood pressure.

CONSIDERATIONS: The oil is slightly photosensitizing.

EMOTIONAL ATTRIBUTE: The sedative fragrance counters depression, hysteria, shock and nervous tension.

Associated Oils:

Bitter Orange (C. *aurantium var. amara*)—Pressed from the peel, bitter orange oil has similar properties to sweet orange. Photosensitizing.

Grapefruit (C. *x paradisi*)—The oil from the peel encourages weight loss and gallbladder activity, and is noted for its cleansing action. It is a favorite of children, and we find it useful for inner-child work. It often accents bergamot.

Lime (C. *aurantiifolia*)—Native to India and Southeast Asia, this is the most tender citrus tree. Unlike other citruses, the peel can be steam-distilled as well as pressed. Lime flavors cola beverages and is used in the treatment of depression.

Tangerine or ***Mandarin*** (C. *reticulata*)—From the peel of mandarin orange, this oil counters insomnia, lymph congestion, fat reduction and digestive problems. It is a safer citrus oil for children and pregnant women.

Orange Blossom (Neroli)
(*Citrus aurantium var. amara*)

One of the many stories about this plant is that neroli was named after the 16th-century Italian princess of Nerola, who loved its scent. The oil comes from the blossom of the bitter orange, not the sweet orange that produces orange oil. An Indochina native, it is grown commercially in France, Morocco, Tunisia and Egypt.

FAMILY: Rutaceae

EXTRACTION: Distilled from blossoms. Concrete, absolute. The fragrance is sweet, spicy and distinctive.

MEDICINAL ACTION: Neroli treats diarrhea and circulation problems such as hemorrhoids and high blood pressure.

COSMETIC/SKIN USE: Used on mature and couperose skin to regenerate the cells.

EMOTIONAL ATTRIBUTE: One of the best aromatic antidepressives, neroli counters emotional shock, mental confusion, nervous strain, anxiety, fear and lack of confidence. It redirects one's energy into a more positive direction, countering both fatigue and insomnia. It is used for those who get upset for no apparent reason. Also an aphrodisiac.

Associated Oils:

Petitgrain (C. *aurantium*)—Now distilled from the fragrant leaves and stems of the bitter orange, this oil originally came from the small, unripe fruit (thus its name, "little fruit"). The fragrance resembles neroli, but is harsher and sharper. It is less expensive and potent, but often effective enough as an antidepressant. Petitgrain increases perception and awareness and reestablishes trust and self-confidence. Most of the oil comes from Paraguay, where the 19th-century French botanist Benjamin Balansa first distilled the leaves.

Neroli Portugal (C. *aurantium var. dulcis*)—The flowers of this sweeter orange produce a less fragrant oil, also called *neroli petalea*, considered inferior to *var. amara*.

Patchouli (*Pogostemon cablin*)

Because the scent is developed by oxidation, the succulent leaves of this pretty East Indian bush carry little indication of their potential. The leaves are aged before being distilled, which takes up to 24 hours. Even then, the oil is harsh. As it ages, the translucent yellow oil turns syrupy brown as it develops patchouli's distinctive fragrance, so popular in the 1960s. Patchouli continues to get better with age. Many people have never smelled the high-quality oil, which is used in famous perfumes such as Tabu and Shocking. The oil comes from Indonesia, India and especially China. An effective pest deterrent, it is used to keep wool moths out of woolen shawls and rugs imported from India. Europeans wouldn't buy the imitation rugs because they didn't smell "authentic" (i.e., of patchouli).

FAMILY: Lamiaceae (Labiatae)

EXTRACTION: Distilled from fermented leaves. The fragrance is heavy, earthy, woody, musty, vanilla-like and most distinctive. Resinoid.

MEDICINAL ACTION: It helps reduce appetite, water retention, exhaustion and inflammation.

COSMETIC/SKIN USE: As a cell rejuvenator and antiseptic, the oil treats acne, eczema, inflamed, cracked or mature skin, and dandruff. As an antifungal, it treats athlete's foot.

EMOTIONAL ATTRIBUTE: Patchouli counters nervousness and depression by putting problems into perspective and releasing pent-up emotions. Though an aphrodisiac, it helps insomnia.

Pepper, Black (*Piper nigrum*)

Pepper is a semitropical climbing shrub from India, where most oil and peppercorns for seasoning are produced. Some also comes from Indonesia and the Orient.

FAMILY: Piperacea

EXTRACTION: Distilled from partially dried, unripe fruit. The scent is spicy, sharp and slightly herbaceous. An oil with a more fruity fragrance is also produced from the fresh green fruit.

MEDICINAL ACTION: Treats food poisoning, indigestion, colds, flu, urinary-tract infections, congested lungs, fevers and poor circulation.

COSMETIC/SKIN USE: On the skin, a warming liniment.

EMOTIONAL ATTRIBUTE: The fragrance is emotionally stimulating and, some say, aphrodisiac.

CONSIDERATIONS: Although nontoxic, black pepper can irritate skin.

Associated Oils:

Litsea (*Litsea cubeba*)—Litsea oil is distilled from small, pepperlike fruits of this member of the laurel family from India and Southeast Asia. In the East, the flowers flavor tea. This relaxant treats indigestion, excessive perspiration and acne. Often called "tropical verbena," litsea is actually unrelated to verbena.

Cubeb (*Piper cubeba*)—A litsea substitute.

California Pepper Tree (*Schinus moule*)—This South American tree is a popular ornamental in California. Used to replace pepper in cooking during World War II, it sometimes also replaces it in perfumery and flavoring. South Americans use the berries medicinally.

Mastic (*Pistacia lentiscus*)—Steam-distilled from oleoresin or resinoid, mastic is very astringent and helpful for hemorrhoids. As a balm, this was an ancient trade item, closely related to the Biblical terebinth.

Peppermint (*Mentha piperita*)

Peppermint self-hybridized, probably in the 17th century. It now grows wild throughout Europe, North America and Australia. After the *British Medical Journal* noted in 1879 that menthol relieves headaches and neuralgia, menthol cones (which evaporate into the air) and scented candles became the rage. Peppermint is one of the few essential-oil plants grown and distilled in the United States where the light cloud cover over central Oregon and Michigan increases the production of oil, most of which is redistilled to produce a lighter mint flavor for candies and gums. Several mints are also distilled for perfumery.

FAMILY: Lamiaceae (Labiatae)

EXTRACTION: Distilled from leaves. Peppermint has a powerful, minty-fresh odor.

MEDICINAL ACTION: Peppermint alleviates digestive-tract spasms, indigestion, nausea, ulcers and irritable-bowel syndrome, and helps destroy bacteria, viruses and parasites in the digestive tract. It also clears sinus and lung congestion, and is used to treat muscle spasms and inflammation.

COSMETIC/SKIN USE: Peppermint stimulates the skin's oil production. It also relieves the itching skin of ringworm, herpes simplex, scabies and poison oak. Because it is warming (especially the oil that isn't redistilled), it is often used in liniments.

EMOTIONAL ATTRIBUTE: As a stimulant, the scent counters insomnia, shock, mental fogginess and lack of focus. It also unblocks "stuck" emotions.

CONSIDERATIONS: Watch out—too much may burn the skin.

Associated Oils:

Spearmint (*M. spicata*)—Somewhat weaker in action, spearmint brings back childhood joy and memories. It is the mint of choice for pregnant women, with fewer irritating and toxic constituents.

Cornmint (*M. arvensis*)—This species is less sweet, but contains much more menthol, making it a good choice for liniments. Cornmint is the source of natural menthol crystals used in liniments and some lipsticks, in hair tonics and in other body-care products to produce a stimulating/cooling sensation. The herb is grown in China and Japan, and also in Brazil by descendants of the Japanese immigrants who introduced it.

Pennyroyal (*M. pulegium*)—The scent and oil are harsher than other mints, so pennyroyal must be used with care and never by pregnant women. It is used occasionally to treat fever, itching skin, indigestion, congestion from colds, scant, painful menstruation and to deter fleas, but it is potentially toxic because of its pulegone content. The scent relieves dizziness—the Romans even wore pennyroyal head garlands to dispel drunkenness. Culpeper dabbed the waters on headaches, the vinegar on bruises and burns. We recommend the much safer herb tea, but even that should be avoided by pregnant women.

Ravensare (*Ravensara aromatica*)

A large tree from Madagascar, where the seeds are a popular spice, ravensare is a personal favorite of ours for any infection.

FAMILY: Lauraceae

EXTRACTION: Distilled from leaves and sometimes from fruit and bark. The scent is similar to eucalyptus, but softer and more refined.

MEDICINAL ACTION: Ravensare is an antiseptic treatment for flu, bronchitis, viral infections, shingles, viral hepatitis and sinus congestion. It also helps relieve muscle fatigue.

COSMETIC/SKIN USE: Useful for acne.

Rose (*Rosa damascena, R. gallica,* and others)

The fragrance of rose has inspired poets and lovers throughout the ages. The Greek poetess Sappho christened it "queen of flowers" in 600 BC. Although originally distilled in Asia Minor, today Bulgaria is the world's largest producer, making the most valued rose oil. Turkey still produces a slightly less expensive oil, although all rose oil is costly, not just because so little is produced during distillation but because the bushes themselves need so much care. It is very nontoxic, and specific for women's problems.

FAMILY: Rosaceae

EXTRACTION: Distilled (rose otto) or solvent extracted (rose absolute) from blossoms. Unlike most essential oils, rose oil is difficult to separate from water because its constituents are very water-soluble, so it is distilled at least twice. The resulting rose otto congeals at cool room temperature because of its natural waxes. Rose water is a by-product of distillation. The fragrance of rose is wonderfully intense, sweet and floral, and it is easily recognized.

MEDICINAL ACTION: Rose treats asthma, hay fever, liver problems, nausea, most female disorders and impotency in men. Tests reveal that it increases the sperm count. "Honey of Red Rose" was recommended for sore mouths and throats in U.S. and British pharmacopoeias.

COSMETIC/SKIN USE: A cell rejuvenator, rose soothes and heals burns and all skin complexion types. It is also strongly antiseptic and fights infection. Although it is nontoxic, strong solutions can irritate the face.

EMOTIONAL ATTRIBUTE: Rose helps alleviate depression and lack of confidence. It has long inspired love and "opens" the heart. Employed for relationship conflicts, envy and intolerance, it is comforting, supportive during crisis and an aphrodisiac.

Associated Oil:

Cabbage Rose (*R. centifolia*)—Also called "rose de mai," this oil is less expensive than its Bulgarian counterpart. Once cultivated extensively in France, cabbage rose now comes mostly from Morocco.

Rosemary (*Rosmarinus officinalis*)

Rosmarinus means "dew of the sea," where this Mediterranean herb loves to grow. Rosemary delights the late winter with prolific blooms. Rosemary was the main ingredient in "Hungary Water" and the first cologne. The old French name *incensier* came from rosemary's celebrated history as church incense. Until the 20th century, the fragrant leaves were burned to purify French hospitals. Commoners burned rosemary instead of frankincense; it symbolized both love and death at funerals.

FAMILY: Lamiaceae (Labiatae)

EXTRACTION: Distilled from flowering tops or leaves. The powerful fragrance is herby, sharp and camphorous.

MEDICINAL ACTION: Rosemary is one of the best stimulants. It also improves poor circulation, lowers cholesterol, eases muscle and rheumatism pains, and treats lung congestion, sore throat and canker sores. It stimulates the nervous system, motor nerves, adrenals and a sluggish gallbladder. It is often used in penetrating liniments.

COSMETIC/SKIN USE: An age-old remedy for dandruff and hair loss, the branches were even used as hair brushes. Rosemary helps sluggish, underactive skin, and is used on dry, mature and couperose skin types. It also helps in the treatment of cellulite and skin parasites.

EMOTIONAL ATTRIBUTE: Rosemary improves memory, confidence, perception and creativity, and helps balance mind and body. It prevents dizziness, dark thoughts and nightmares (and helps you remember the good dreams). The smoke was inhaled for brain weakness. (As Shakespeare said, "There's rosemary, that's for remembrance . . . ")

CONSIDERATIONS: Rosemary can overstimulate, and may increase blood pressure.

Associated Oils:

Rosemarinus officinalis has several chemotypes:

Borneol type—Helps overcome fatigue and infections, and is a heart tonic.

Camphor type—A vein decongestant, mucolytic, cardiac tonic and diuretic.

Cineol type—For lung congestion, cystitis and chronic fatigue.

Verbenone type—Mucolytic, sinus infections, antispasmodic, and helps balance the endocrine and nervous systems. For oily or regenerative skin care, but contains some potentially hazardous ketones.

Rosmarinus Pyramidalis (R. pyramidalis)—This has respiratory applications, but is specific for ear and sinus problems.

Rosewood (*Aniba rosaeodora*)

The French call this South American rain forest tree *bois de rose*, or "wood of rose." Rosewood was first distilled in 1875 in French Guiana, but became so popular that the trees were all cut. It is one of the many plants that make the rain forest a valuable resource to be protected, but it is also one that promotes their destruction. We hope that what happened in French Guiana will not be repeated, and recommend using rose geranium as a substitute.

FAMILY: Lauraceae

EXTRACTION: Distilled from wood chips. The pleasant fragrance is sweet, woodsy and rosy.

MEDICINAL ACTION: Eases headaches, cold, fever, infections, vaginitis and nausea.

COSMETIC/SKIN USE: Rejuvenates cells and helps all skin types.

EMOTIONAL ATTRIBUTE: An antidepressant, rosewood encourages tranquility and constructive emotional work.

Sage (*Salvia officinalis*)

Familiar as a culinary herb, sage comes from Spain and Asia Minor. In medieval times it was used as a nervous-system tonic to reduce tics or epilepsy. Because its essential oil has antioxidant properties, the herb was used to preserve food. In ancient Crete, the burning leaves were inhaled to relieve asthma. Only a few of the many sage species are distilled. We've made wonderful hydrosol from some of the rare ones, such as pineapple sage.

FAMILY: Lamiaceae (Labiatae)

EXTRACTION: Distilled from leaves. The odor is spicy, sharp and very herby. An oleoresin is produced from the exhausted material.

MEDICINAL ACTION: Sage, a decongestant with strong antiseptic properties, treats throat and mouth infections. It also has hormonal action (estrogenic), regulating the menstrual cycle, decreasing lactation and alleviating menopause symptoms.

COSMETIC/SKIN USE: Reduces perspiration, oily skin, and acne, and is said to encourage hair growth.

EMOTIONAL ATTRIBUTE: Sage helps those suffering from nervous debility, excessive sexual desire, grief, physical overexertion and insomnia. It encourages "inward focus." Gerard said of sage, "It is singularly good for the head, brain . . . it quickeneth the senses, memory."

CONSIDERATIONS: Contains thujone, a neurotoxic ketone, so avoid this oil for anyone prone to seizures. Sage is harsh and irritating on the skin, so use low dilutions.

Associated Oil:

Spanish Sage (*S. lavandulaefolia*)—Less toxic and irritating than common sage. The distinctive lavender fragrance is so strong it is often mistaken for lavender. Use for acne, eczema and dermatitis, or to help relieve arthritis, poor circulation and the flu.
(Also see *clary sage*.)

Sandalwood (*Santalum album*)

One of the oldest perfume materials, sandalwood has been in use for at least 2,000 years. It begins producing oil only after 30 years. Mysore, India, produces the best-quality oil, which is regulated by the government, but oil is also available from Indonesia. Australia distills the inferior *S. spicatum*.

FAMILY: Santalaceae

EXTRACTION: Distilled from heartwood and roots. The scent is balsamic, soft, warm and woody.

MEDICINAL ACTION: Once a gonorrhea treatment, sandalwood is still used for genital and urinary infections. It also counters inflammation, hemorrhoids, persistent coughs, nausea, throat problems and some types of nerve pain. It is nontoxic.

COSMETIC/SKIN USE: Suitable for all complexion types, sandalwood is especially useful on rashes, inflammation, and dry acne or chapped skin.

EMOTIONAL ATTRIBUTE: Depression, anxiety and insomnia are improved by sandalwood. It helps promote spiritual practices, peaceful relaxation, openness and "grounding." It is used in death ceremonies to help the soul cross over, and to comfort mourners.

Associated Oil:

Amyris (*Amyris balsamifera*)—This small Haitian tree, called "West Indian rosewood," often adulterates or replaces sandalwood, especially in so-called "sandalwood" soaps.

Spikenard (*Nardostachys jatamansi*)

Mentioned in the Bible in the Song of Solomon, spikenard was used by the ancient Egyptians and the Romans for *nardinum* ointment. Spikenard is the same heady oil lavishly poured over the feet of Christ by Mary Magdalene. It remains very expensive.

FAMILY: Valerianaceae

EXTRACTION: Distilled from rhizome. The scent is earthy and strong, reminiscent of both valerian and patchouli.

MEDICINAL ACTION: Treats nervous indigestion, insomnia, headache, hemorrhoids and heart palpitations.

COSMETIC/SKIN USE: Use spikenard for inflammation, dry or mature complexion, rashes and psoriasis.

EMOTIONAL ATTRIBUTE: Spikenard relieves emotional tension and insomnia.

Associated Oils:

Valerian (*Valeriana officinalis*)—Isovaleric acid is responsible for a strong and pungent odor that has been compared to dirty socks. Like the herb, the oil is sedating. It is grown in the Baltic states, in Belgium and in Germany. There is also an Indian valerian (*V. wallichii*).

Kesso Root (*V. officinalis var. latifolia*)—This Japanese variety is sometimes aged to increase the strong odor.

Tea Tree (*Melaleuca alternifolia*)

This large Australian tree, sometimes also spelled "ti," is related to eucalyptus. There are many species and subspecies; all have an interesting bark that curls off the trunk, giving them the name "paperbark." Studies show that contact with blood and pus actually increases tea tree's antiseptic powers. The scents are easier to distinguish when the fresh leaves of different species are being crushed than after the oil has been distilled, and we suspect that with so many different species, the oils aren't always properly identified. Tea tree is nontoxic, with uses as wide-ranging as those of lavender.

FAMILY: Myrtaceae

EXTRACTION: Distilled from leaves. The scent is similar to eucalyptus, but softer. Poor-quality oil smells like melted rubber.

MEDICINAL ACTION: A good immune-system tonic, tea tree fights lung, genital and urinary, vaginal, sinus and mouth infections. It counters fungal infections and viral infections such as herpes, shingles, chicken pox, candida, thrush and flu.

COSMETIC/SKIN USE: Tea tree treats diaper rash, fungus, acne, wounds and insect bites. It protects the skin from radiation burns during cancer therapy. It is one of the most nonirritating antiseptic oils, although this varies with the species.

EMOTIONAL ATTRIBUTE: The scent builds strength, especially before an operation and during postoperative shock.

Associated Oils:

Cajeput (*M. cajuputii*)—The name comes from the Malaysian *caju-puti*, meaning "white bark." It is a vein decongestant and is harsher than tea tree oil.

M. quinquenervia—This is a sweeter-smelling species of tea tree. The commercially sold "MQV" is a type of this oil.

Niaouli (*M. viridiflora*)—Called "Gomen oil" because it was once shipped from that West Indies port, Niaouli is now harvested in Australia. The antiviral properties are similar to those of tea tree, but is considered more effective fighting viruses such as herpes, and has a sweeter, more pleasant fragrance.

Thyme (*Thymus vulgaris*)

Rudyard Kipling wrote of the "wind-bit thyme that smells like the perfume of the dawn in paradise." Ancient Greeks complimented each other as "smelling like *thymbra*"; their word *thymain* meant "to burn as incense," and *thymiatechny* described the "art of using perfumes as medicine." The compound thymol is still used in gargles such as Listerine, in cough drops and in vapor rubs. There are at least a hundred varieties (or double that if you count the cultivars.)

FAMILY: Lamiaceae (Labiatae)

EXTRACTION: Distilled from leaves. Absolute. The scent is strong, herbaceous, sweet and medicinal.

MEDICINAL ACTION: Thyme is a strong antibacterial for mouth infections. It relieves lung congestion, treats candida and indigestion, and destroys intestinal hookworms and roundworms. It is used in a heating liniment, and was once a specific remedy for whooping cough.

EMOTIONAL ATTRIBUTE: Thyme relieves mental instability, melancholy and nightmares, and prevents memory loss and inefficiency.

Associated Oils:

Thymus vulgaris has many chemotypes:

Geraniol Type—This gentle antiseptic treats vaginitis, cystitis, acne, eczema and earache. It is a uterine and cardiac tonic with mildness comparable to linalol.

Linalol Type—This is a nontoxic antiseptic useful in the treatment of candida, bronchitis, acne, nervous fatigue, psoriasis, urinary tract infections and prostate problems. Linalol is nonirritating, so it is gentle enough for children and skin care.

Red Thyme (*T. vulgaris*)—This is oil that hasn't been redistilled, so it retains a deep red color. Hotter and more irritating than distilled thyme, it is a strong infection fighter and circulatory stimulant.

Thymol Type—Stimulating and very antibacterial, this thyme is also irritating to skin and mucous membranes.

Thuyanol Type—This type is high in thuyanol and terpenes, but low in the more toxic phenols. A nonirritating antiseptic, it treats viral infections, and French research shows it effective against chlamydia, condyloma and many female infections.

White Thyme (*T. vulgaris*)—This has been redistilled, yielding a clear oil. It is somewhat less irritating and potent than "red thyme" oil.

Moroccan Thyme (*T. satureioides*)—Sometimes referred to as "sweet thyme," this species contains 70-80 percent borneal, an immune-supporting alcohol. It is a digestive stimulant, settles the nerves, and is used to treat Chronic Fatigue Syndrome.

Spanish Marjoram *(T. mastichina)*—See "Marjoram."

Spanish Oregano *(T. capitatus)*—See "Marjoram."

Tuberose (*Polianthes tuberosa*)

One of the most expensive of the flower oils, this intensely fragrant Mexican flower has found international fame in perfumes such as White Shoulders and Chloe. The Aztecs prized tuberose for medicine. Hawaiian leis are often made with it. The name describes its tuberous root.

FAMILY: Agavaceae

EXTRACTION: In the past, enfleurage of flower. (The *absolute d'enfleurage* has a fatty note due to small residues of lard.) The solvent-extracted oil has a slightly "green" scent. Concrete. Absolute. The odor is floral, very sweet and honeylike, with a hint of camphor. Sometimes the oil is made from the slightly less odorous double-petaled garden flower.

EMOTIONAL ATTRIBUTE: The fragrance is sensual and aphrodisiac. Its East Indian name, *rat ki rani*, means "mistress of the night."

Vanilla (*Vanilla planifolia*)

This tropical flower, an orchid, is a Mexican native grown in Tahiti, Java and Madagascar. Orchids are considered the most highly evolved flowers, and this is the only one with an edible fruit. When first transplanted in Réunion, vanilla didn't produce pods because the hummingbirds and bees that pollinate it didn't live there. A hand-pollination method developed in 1841 is still used today.

FAMILY: Orchidaceae

EXTRACTION: Resinoid, absolute, oleoresin, CO_2. The scent is sweet, "creamy" and typically vanilla.

EMOTIONAL ATTRIBUTE: Vanilla's fragrance improves one's confidence and helps to dissolve pent-up anger and frustration. It is consoling and can unleash hidden, often subconscious, sensuality.

Vetiver (*Vetiveria zizanoides*)

Not a picturesque plant with its grasslike leaves, vetiver's (or vetivert) thin, aromatic roots are its treasure. They are distilled in Java, Réunion, Haiti, Brazil and India. Door and window screens (called *tatties*) and fans are woven in East India from the spindly roots. The British occupation of India made vetiver waters and colognes popular in 19th-century England and North America. The perfume *Mousseline des Indes* took its name from Indian muslin that was scented with vetiver to protect it from insects. Two other Victorian perfumes, *Maréchale* and *Bouquet de Roi*, were also based on vetiver. Modern perfumes use it as a fixative.

FAMILY: Gramineae

EXTRACTION: Distilled from the root. It has an earthy, heavy scent. An inferior oil is made from used vetiver screens.

MEDICINAL ACTION: Vetiver eases muscular pain, sprains and liver congestion, and is a circulatory stimulant.

COSMETIC/SKIN USE: Vetiver treats acne, wounds and dry skin.

EMOTIONAL ATTRIBUTE: The scent is uplifting, relaxing, and comforting, releasing deep fears and tensions. It cools the body and mind of excessive heat.

Violet (*Viola odorata*)

The fragrance temporarily makes you lose your sense of smell, leading Shakespeare to muse, "The perfume, suppliance of a minute. No more." Medieval patients drank violet water; they were rubbed with violet oil, then wrapped in linen. Romans splashed violet vinegar on headaches. In the 19th century, French perfumer Charles Piesse said violets were so popular the demand was more than he could supply. Some oil is produced in France and Italy, but most comes from Egypt.

FAMILY: Violaceae

EXTRACTION: Absolute, concrete from leaves, rarely flowers. The leaf odor is green, leafy and peppery.

EMOTIONAL ATTRIBUTE: The fragrance helps one realize potential and dissipate confusion, nervous exhaustion and insomnia. It was once said to comfort and strengthen the heart.

Associated Oil:

Orris *(Iris germanica var. florentina)*—Orris essential oil often replaced violet as a less expensive scent, but at the current $25,000 a pound, it is no longer a cheap alternative. Before distilling, the peeled roots must be aged two years to develop their scent. The main growers are Tuscany and Morocco.

Yarrow (*Achillea millefolium*)

This common herb is found in temperate climates around the world. The blue calming azulene is created during distillation, although some yarrow oils lack azulene and, therefore, the color.

FAMILY: Asteraceae (Compositae)

EXTRACTION: Distilled from herb and flowers. The odor is green, herbaceous and sharp.

MEDICINAL ACTION: Yarrow treats digestive and muscular cramps, hemorrhoids, menstrual irregularity and urinary infections.

COSMETIC/SKIN USE: Helps heal rashes and wounds, acne, eczema, inflammation, varicose veins, and wounds. It is also used as a hair tonic.

EMOTIONAL ATTRIBUTE: Yarrow instills a sense of security and assists long-range planning.

Ylang-Ylang (*Cananga odorata*)

Ylang-ylang means "flower of flowers." The trees, bearing fragrant drooping yellow flowers, are grown for the perfume trade in Réunion. The oil varies greatly because of climatic and botanical differences. The four commercial grades are: Extra (the finest, first distillation), One, Two and Three. There is also the less expensive cananga oil, with an inferior scent. Rich in terpenes and low in esters.

FAMILY: Annonaceae

EXTRACTION: Distilled from flowers. The intensely sweet odor is heady (described by some as bananalike) and floral. Absolute, concrete.

MEDICINAL ACTION: A strong sedative, ylang-ylang is antispasmodic and helps lower blood pressure.

COSMETIC/SKIN USE: Used as a hair tonic and to balance oil production in all skin types, although most often recommended for oily and problem skin.

EMOTIONAL ATTRIBUTE: The fragrance makes the senses more acute and tempers depression, fear, jealousy, anger and frustration. It is aphrodisiac in low doses.

CONSIDERATIONS: High concentrations can produce headaches or nausea.

Associated Oils:

Champac *(Michelia champaca)*—From Indonesia and India, this heady scent is quite expensive, so it is sometimes adulterated with ylang-ylang. It has long been extracted into vegetable oil. Today it is mostly cultivated in the Philippines and is available as a concrete and absolute.

Cananga *(type macrophylla)*—Rich in terpenes and low in esters, this oil has an inferior scent.

7

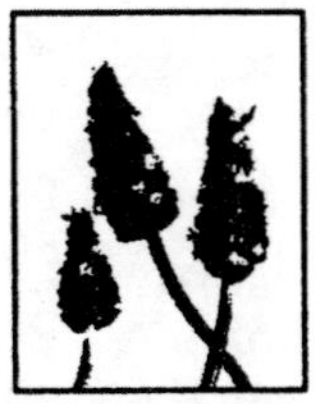

Aromatherapy Massage

The way to health is to have an aromatic bath and a scented massage every day.

—Hippocrates

Aromatherapy enhances any type of body work by positively influencing the subject's moods and increasing relaxation. Essential oils are absorbed through the skin into the blood system for therapeutic actions, so simply rubbing the body oil into the skin directly over the problem—say, an upset stomach or headache—puts the oil right where it is needed.

If you've ever given a massage, you know that it often takes the person receiving the treatment some time to relax fully. Slowly, but very slowly, the breathing slows down and deepens. Tense muscles begin to relax. When you use an aromatherapy massage oil, you will be surprised how quickly the person slips into deep relaxation states that usually take at least an hour of massage to achieve. The longer you work, the deeper he or she goes.

As professional masseuses we have had wonderful experiences using the two techniques together, but don't think that you must be a trained masseuse or masseur to qualify to use body oils with massage. Even if you aren't familiar with massage techniques, you can still give a therapeutic rub that will make the recipient feel good. You can even treat yourself to a massage: you may want to rub your own tight shoulders or cellulite thighs twice daily with aromatherapy oils.

Among the best oils to relieve stress and muscle pain are bergamot, clary sage, chamomile, jasmine, lavender, marjoram, neroli, rose, rosemary, sandalwood and ylang-ylang. Liniments made with warming oils such as peppermint, cinnamon and cloves relieve or inhibit muscle soreness. Oils can also be specifically designed for foot massage, for babies, for headache relief, for pregnant women, even for helping reduce cellulite. We've provided a variety of simple formulas to get you started.

For any type of massage, make sure that the oils are lightly fragranced. Too strong a smell quickly overwhelms both the person getting and the one giving the massage. The most therapeutic action occurs when the scent is very faint, just barely detectable. (You'll find people actually liking lighter versions of oils they otherwise wouldn't care for.) We suggest a two-percent dilution of essential oil in a carrier oil for a standard massage oil. When doing a lymph-drainage massage, or other type of body work requiring lots of massage oil, lower dilutions may be more appropriate. For a liniment, which must be more concentrated to work properly, a three-percent dilution is generally sufficient.

If you are working as a professional, you will need a well-ventilated room: otherwise, by the third client of the day you'll be dizzy from all the oils. Nothing fancy is needed; airing out the room between clients by opening the windows or using a fan is usually sufficient. If that's not possible, use an air filter to remove scent from the air. Monitor the room to check how strong it smells: walk outside, stroll around, take a few deep breaths, then come back inside. You may be surprised how accustomed you've become to the scent and how strong the room really smells.

Essential oils are versatile and can treat many common problems. Ideally, oil blends are custom-designed for individuals. This demands some skill in blending—this book's "Blending" chapter should be enough to start you out—and some skill in choosing the most appropriate oils. Until you have enough expertise, stick to simple problems and focus on relaxation, which is healing in itself. Custom blending is beneficial if you have the time, but not always necessary.

We like to keep a selection of aromatherapy body oils on hand to treat the most common complaints. If you're going to be doing much body work, make a series of blends. Use the various charts in this book for ideas on designing body oils for individual needs.

LEGAL IMPLICATIONS AND SAFETY PRECAUTIONS

In the United States, certified body workers are allowed to give a relaxing massage, but treating internal problems steps beyond the boundaries of the law. However, you may give specific treatments to your family and friends. Professional body workers may give an aromatherapy massage treatment as long as they are just providing relaxation, instead of diagnosing and treating physical or emotional disorders. Just keep a few safety precautions in mind:

- Don't treat beyond your scope of knowledge.
- Make pleasing aromatherapy blends, not medicinal formulas.
- Use words such as "balance," "nourish," "assist," "tone," "uplift" and "relax."
- Don't try to come up with a medical "diagnosis" or "prescribe."
- Know when and where to refer those with severe problems.
- Don't massage strenuously near varicose veins, bruises or other types of broken veins.
- Watch out for sensitivities to the essential oils.

EXTRA TOUCHES

There are many ways to incorporate aromatherapy into a massage treatment. Most people enjoy being pampered, especially when they are getting a massage. All of the extra touches make the massage you give special. Lightly misting a floral water or hydrosol over the person receiving the massage gives a special touch to any type of body work. Just be sure to do it high enough in the air so that droplets don't chill the subject's skin.

To relax a person before you begin a massage, place a warm herbal compress over tight muscles. Simply add a few drops of an appropriate essential oil to very warm water. Any of the essential oils suggested for massage are suitable for a compress. Submerge a soft cloth into the water, swish it around, wring it out and place it on the skin for two to five minutes, or even longer if you have time—just don't let the cloth cool and become uncomfortable. For an extended treatment, place a towel or a heating pad over the compress to keep it warm. After removing the compress, pat the skin dry with a warm towel.

A compress over the eyes, either before or after a massage, is very relaxing and relieves headache. Use gentle oils such as chamomile and be sure to dilute well; avoid hot oils such as peppermint, clove and cinnamon, which can burn delicate eyelids. (Be sure to never put essential oils *in* your eyes.) You can also use hydrosols as an eye compress or to gently mist the face.

SPECIAL TYPES OF MASSAGE

Aromatherapy can be used in other types of body work and special types of massage. For acupressure or other methods that don't normally use a massage oil, a small amount of oil can safely be applied to the fingertips. The massage oil can be used with or without acupressure to "spot" and activate certain areas. Other methods of aromatherapy, such as an essential oil diffuser or a potpourri cooker filled with water, can be used in body work that does not require body oil. A few drops of essential oil will fill the room with fragrance.

Cellulite Massage

Cellulite, really just a fancy word for puckered fat, has been characterized as "orange-peel skin" (textured and lumpy), and is found most often in the thighs and buttocks. Cellulite affects women more than men and does not necessarily result from overweight. The following formula, used in a bath or as a massage oil, is most effective if combined with other weight-loss activities, such as restricting dietary fat and exercising. Geranium and fennel are hormone balancers which, with grapefruit, have historically been used to facilitate weight loss. Cypress and juniper stimulate circulation, and juniper is a diuretic.

Cellulite Formula

10 drops cypress oil
10 drops geranium oil
10 drops grapefruit oil
5 drops juniper oil
5 drops fennel oil
4 ounces carrier oil

Pregnancy Massage

A pregnant woman's expanding belly needs massage and aromatherapy oils to help the skin expand and thus prevent stretch marks. To massage a pregnant woman, support her with pillows to make her as comfortable as possible, and select only the safest essential oils (see "Guidelines" chapter). The important consideration is that she be comfortable, not strained or compressed anywhere. If lying down is impractical or uncomfortable, she can sit facing the back of a straight chair for a back massage. Common sense and thoughtfulness are really all you'll need. Apply the appropriate oil to the belly at least twice a day. The following belly-oil formula is suitable for the whole body. A pregnant woman probably will also want her lower back massaged. Although it's always a pleasure to have someone else give you a massage, fortunately the belly is in a handy location for self-massage. If you want to use an oil infused with herbs as the carrier oil, a good choice is calendula flower. A belly oil is ideal for giving a new mom a massage after birth. Add a couple drops of clary sage to help counter postpartum depression.

Many women also appreciate some massaging during labor to promote relaxation. Lavender is an old standby in the birthing room. As mentioned in our "Scent and Psyche" chapter, lavender flowers traditionally were heated, pounded into a poultice, then placed on the woman's lower back. Lavender was chosen because it is a muscle relaxant that "opens up" constricted areas. Old texts talk of its ability to "raise the spirit" of the people attending the birth, and also to "raise the spirit" of the child who is coming into the world.

It would be nice to see lavender returned to the birthing room, even though poultices are messy to make and use, especially during birth when a pregnant woman is likely to be changing positions. The perfect alternative is a lavender massage oil, such as the Pregnant-Belly Oil described below, which can be rubbed into a tight back or anywhere the woman feels tension. The light scent imparted into the air will serve the ancient purpose of raising the spirit even better than a poultice.

Oil for a Pregnant Belly

15 drops lavender oil
5 drops neroli oil
2 drops rose oil
4 ounces carrier oil (Calendula is good)
800 IU vitamin E

Rose and neroli are both expensive, so make this oil with just lavender if you wish.

Muscle Massage

Everyone has at least a few tight muscles. The shoulders and neck are favorite places for storing tension, but muscles anywhere in the body can become cramped. Muscle cramping, including menstrual cramps, is greatly relieved by massage with a muscle-relaxing massage oil. You may not think that stomachaches and gas pains need external treatment, but these problems are generally caused by muscle cramping and are thus helped by gentle massage. Similarly, rubbing massage oil on the temples helps relieve a tension headache.

Muscle Massage Oil

30 drops lavender oil
10 drops marjoram oil
5 drops clary sage oil
2 ounces carrier oil

Facial Massage

Did you know that more muscles are concentrated in your face than anywhere else in your body? These muscles allow you to smile, cry and pout, but all of that movement leads to some very tired face muscles. Facial tension contributes to wrinkles and to poor blood circulation in your face.

A facial massage makes a good accompaniment to the aromatherapy facial described in the "Facial Care" chapter. It's also a very nice way to introduce someone to massage. (A good facial massage takes much less time than a body massage.) Always use very lightly scented oils around the face, and be sure to keep oil well away from the eyes. We recommend a 2-percent dilution. Go light on the amount of oil as well. Often a thick facial cream works best.

A good sequence for a facial massage is to begin at the chin and work up, against gravity. If there's time, give the tight shoulders and neck a quick rub. Be sure to use gentle, light strokes on the face—kneading the face too much only contributes to more wrinkling. Because you're working on such a small area with so many different planes, tiny circular motions are good for most of the face. A light tapping motion with the fingers, as though you're typing, gives a stimulating massage without being at all abrasive. Don't forget to work around the ears and the jaws, areas that frequently hold tension.

Baby Massage

Most babies love massage, and they are very expressive, so it's easy to tell what a baby likes and dislikes. Listen and observe them, and use this as your guide to the amount of pressure (begin very gently) and the best types of strokes. Baby massages tend to be short. Watch for a response; when the baby begins getting fussy or bored, it's time to stop.

You don't need many guidelines, and you certainly don't need to know any fancy strokes to simply rub in an oil. Do make sure, however, that your hands aren't too rough (or your nails too long) for the child's tender skin. Also, avoid putting oil on the baby's hands or face, because it can easily get into the eyes. (Babies tend to dislike a face massage anyway.)

In Europe, massage is widely used as a treatment for colic. Colic is caused by stress and indigestion, two of the problems helped most by massage. In the late 1980s, the clinic of the Danish physician Jan-Helge Larson prescribed belly massage for colicky babies. Support the baby under the arms, and place one hand under the stomach. Starting at the navel, use that hand to work in a clockwise direction around the abdomen for at least 15 minutes after a feeding. This helps expel the gas pains that result in colic. It's easiest to sit down to do this massage, although you may want to do it while walking and gently swinging the baby if he or she needs to be calmed.

Another colic-relief method is to lay the baby on its back, gently rotate the legs, then massage the belly. Don't try this right after feeding, because this position makes burping difficult, and insufficient burping contributes to colic. Of course, even a baby who doesn't have colic will still appreciate the massage.

Massage isn't just for babies. Older children will enjoy a massage with baby oil (providing, of course, you give it another name). Because essential oils are absorbed through the skin, massage oils treat problem areas without children having to swallow anything. Ask your little patient what feels good and how hard to press. Most children prefer gentle, light strokes, but not too light—some kids are *very* ticklish.

Baby oil is designed to protect the skin and, of course, to give baby an enjoyable and relaxing massage. Babies are new to our environment, so ingredients that appear mild to us sometimes cause reactions on their delicate skin.

The best baby-care products are made with pure, natural ingredients. Avoid standard commercial baby oil and ointments, which are typically made from mineral oil (petroleum), a good machinery lubricant but questionable for use on skin. Vitamin E (800 IUs) can be added for its skin-healing properties. For a source of vitamin E, pop open a few vitamin capsules. The following formula is an extra-gentle 1-percent dilution.

Herbal Baby Oil

10 drops lavender
4 drops Roman chamomile
4 ounces carrier oil (Calendula oil is good)

Tummy-Rub Oil

6 drops melissa
1 drop chamomile
1 drop fennel oil
2 ounces vegetable oil

Mix ingredients. Rub on every hour or as needed. You can use lavender instead of melissa, which is quite expensive.

Spot Massage and Liniments

Spot massages, using liniments, are good for particularly painful areas. Liniments are used externally to warm or to reduce inflammation, and as disinfectants for spot treatments on wounds or pimples.

Liniments reduce muscle and joint pain. Like body oils they are rubbed into the skin, but contain a higher concentration of warming essential oils, which are potentially irritating. (Use no more than a 3-percent dilution; the idea is to warm the skin, not burn it.) Liniments are designed for spot massage on particularly painful areas, not for an overall body massage. Fitness experts currently suggest applying a liniment before exercise, not afterwards. The liniment's warming action is like a mini-warm-up, relaxing "cold" muscles and allowing them to stretch better. Warm-ups are still a good idea, but you will get a lot more out of them when you use a liniment.

Liniments perform two functions. Primarily, they are heating agents that warm the skin over the muscles or joints. This actually plays a trick on the brain. The brain registers "heat" equals "burning" equals "major problem," and concentrates its attention on the skin's surface, where it senses a potential emergency, instead of on the painful muscle. This breaks the cycle between brain and pain, whereby the painful muscle says, "Oh, this really hurts," and the brain confirms that by signaling pain responses, such as further tightening. With the liniment the focus switches to a dialogue between the perceived "burning" skin and the brain. Thus the painful muscle has a chance to relax while the brain worries about the skin burning.

A liniment may also have a penetrating action, depending on which essential oils you choose. Liniments containing actual muscle-relaxing essential oils, such as rosemary, marjoram and lavender, penetrate the skin to work directly on the muscle. If you prefer, you can make a penetrating liniment that does not heat up the skin.

Now that you understand the principles behind liniments, you are ready to choose the best carrier. Add a 3-percent dilution of essential oils to either vodka (if using rubbing alcohol, which is toxic internally, mark the solution "for external use only") or vegetable oil. Both work fine. The difference between them is that the alcohol emphasizes the cooling nature of the liniment, then quickly evaporates, leaving the essential oils to penetrate the skin. It does not leave any oily residue. On the other hand, because an oil-based liniment stays on the skin, it heats up faster. Oil-based products are easier to massage into the skin, although they leave an oily residue. You can even get fancy and mix alcohol and oil together. Just be sure to shake the mixture before using.

To make an herb-infused liniment, follow the directions for making a tincture or an oil. Generally, this type of oil isn't hot enough by itself, but infused vegetable oil or alcohol can be used as the carrier base, followed by the addition of essential oils.

Liniment Formula

2 ounces carrier oil or alcohol (either rubbing or vodka)
12 drops eucalyptus oil
12 drops peppermint oil
6 drops ginger oil
6 drops cinnamon oil

Mix ingredients. Shake or stir a few times per day for three days to disperse the essential oils in the alcohol.

THE AROMATHERAPY MASSAGE: KATHI'S STORY

My interest in aromatherapy many years ago was sparked by my massage practice.

I was fortunate to be living on an herb farm. As I led tours through the fragrant herb garden, I noticed that each patch produced a different reaction in the visitors. Most interesting was that each group responded again and again in the same way to certain plants. Passing by the rows of lavender always resulted in smiles and raised voices, which dropped as the group approached the chamomile bed. Mint never failed to liven things up again; visitors would begin talking excitedly as they sniffed the pungent leaves. And the honeysuckle—ah, the honeysuckle. Its fragrance found us all reminiscing. I guessed that the source of their reactions was the herb's fragrance, and imagined how I might transfer the reaction onto the massage table.

Lavender seemed a logical beginning because it initiated the strongest responses and was already my favorite. So I cut a handful of its fragrant flowers, placed them in a canning jar and covered them with almond oil. After a few days in the sun, the almond oil in the jar smelled strongly of the lavender, so I strained out the flowers. I awaited my next massage client with a bottle of lavender massage oil close at hand. Because this was the early 1970s and I hadn't heard the term "aromatherapy," I asked if the client would like a "fragrant therapy" massage. Of course, the response was positive. I'm sure the client wasn't sure what I meant, but it sounded pleasant enough to try. That massage, more than 20 years ago, was my initiation into a journey of using fragrance for healing.

My first experiment proved so successful that I couldn't wait to give my next massage. The lavender massages sent the clients into deep relaxation faster than massage alone. At the same time, it soothed sore muscles and headaches, and also seemed to produce a sense of peacefulness. Certainly this was the perfect massage oil, but I couldn't resist exploring other fragrant plants in my herb garden. I found that peppermint gave a spark to anyone who felt exhausted after a long day, that chamomile revived the depressed, and that, yes, the wonderfully fragrant honeysuckle stimulated happy recollections.

I then began to blend different fragrant oils. This proved easier than I had imagined, because I possessed a good nose for fragrance-combining. I was happy to find that as long as the smell was pleasant, the fragrances harmonized. Thus, a relaxing chamomile could blend with a touch of spearmint and the client would feel both relaxed and revitalized.

I produced my first commercial aromatherapy oil in 1975: Herbal Blossom Calming Massage Oil. It contained infused lavender flowers, chamomile flowers and rose petals in almond oil. It was soon followed by a spicy Warm Glow Stimulating Massage Oil of cinnamon, orange and peppermint. Now that I look back on these first formulas, I realize they were quite simple, but they certainly worked well.

The next step was to create body oils from the essential oils themselves. Good-quality essential oils were not so readily available then, but I found some sources and began building up a collection. After much experimentation, I developed seven generic blends so I could offer my massage clients a selection from which to choose.

To do this, I had to ask clients how they were feeling before initiating the massage. I quickly learned the importance of qualifying this request, because my intention was to give an aromatherapy massage, not to listen to a litany of problems. I also asked my clients to take a sniff before I applied the oil. This request might seem simple, but many people are too polite to criticize your creation, especially after you choose it especially for them.

I began then to custom-design oils for each client. First, I would take into consideration the client's brief description of his or her emotional and physical state. Then, as the client prepared for the massage, I quickly blended something special just for the occasion. (My good nose and years of working with fragrant plants came in handy.) I had a selection of about 40 different essential oils from which to choose. The oils were added to a base that I had already prepared by mixing several of my favorite vegetable oils. If the preparation took a few extra minutes, no one minded. After all, what a treat to be massaged with your own personal blend, designed for that moment in time. Truly this was the ultimate aromatherapy massage.

Today, when the massage is complete, I offer a bottle of the client's own special blend to take home for use as bath oil. I also suggest that the client bathe as often as possible to recreate the memory of the relaxation achieved during massage. If it is possible to take an aromatherapy bath just before coming for the next appointment, it will send the client halfway into deep relaxation even before the massage begins.

8

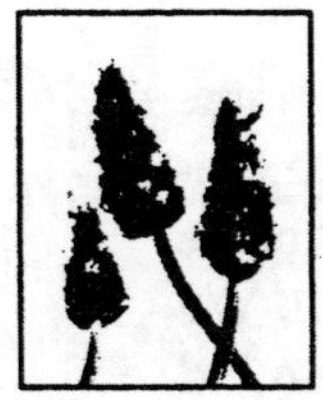

Aromatherapy Body Care

The condition of our hair and skin reflects our inner health and beauty. Nature's gifts of herbs and essential oils offer many benefits for body care. Only a couple of generations ago, women made their own natural products to keep their skin and hair healthy, using common ingredients from recipes handed down through generations.

THE AROMATIC BATH

We can't think of a better way to enjoy the therapeutic benefits of essential oils. Aromatic baths help insomnia, colds, premenstrual syndrome, muscular aches and anxiety—while the warm water promotes additional relaxation.

Essential oils can be added to the bath in undiluted drops, but they are typically hydrophobic (they don't dissolve in water) and lipophilic (drawn to oil). In the bath, therefore, where the only oil medium is your skin, undiluted essential oils are drawn into your body much more quickly than those diluted in a vegetable-oil base. Hot water also causes your skin to be especially receptive to absorbing essential oils. We recommend that you use 3 to 15 drops of essential oil per tub, depending on the particular oils selected and the bather's skin sensitivity.

Oils that are very irritating or stimulating, such as basil, lemongrass, citruses and peppermint, are better mixed in minute amounts with other essential oils in a bath-oil formula than used alone. With nonirritating oils such as lavender, tea tree and geranium, 15 drops are safe as well as delightful.

Some essential oils will disperse on the surface of the water, but many oils will remain in little droplets on top of the water. For best results, fill the tub with water and add the oils just before you get in. Be sure to agitate the water well to distribute the oils. If you do experience any skin irritation in the bath, get out of the tub, rinse with cool water and apply straight vegetable oil to the skin.

Floating Aromatic Bath Oils

Floating aromatic bath oils are wonderful! While bathing, you receive an aromatherapy fragrance treatment, and when you get out, your entire body will be lightly coated with a fragrance that will waft around you for hours. The vegetable-oil base dilutes the essential oil, and helps it to disperse and float over the surface of the water. As you emerge, the oils cling to your skin, scenting it like a body perfume.

Have you ever noticed how your skin shrivels up like a prune after you have been in the water for a long time? The surrounding water actually draws moisture out of your skin. It is loss of water, more than loss of oil, that makes skin feel dry. If you have dry skin, or love to take long soaks in a hot bath, be sure to use an aromatic bath oil. Some people with very dry skin find they can't take baths because their skin itches and feels drier afterward. Their problems will probably disappear when they use an aromatic bath oil, especially one formulated with essential oils suited for this condition, such as sandalwood.

Although an aromatic bath oil may seem like some exotic fragrant concoction, it is extremely easy to create and makes a wonderful aromatherapy gift. It is made by simply diluting essential oils with vegetable oil. We recommend a 4-percent dilution in oil. (Keep in mind that this dilution represents all of the oils in the blend combined, not 4-percent of each oil.) This is double the strength of a massage oil. Add one teaspoon of the bath oil to the water.

Try some blends from our suggested aromatic combinations, listed later in this chapter, for the bath. If you feel creative, make your own combinations. With information from the "Blending" and "Materia Medica" chapters, you can enhance your bath oil with herbs and treat special problems.

An aromatic bath is a perfect way to slow children down, especially at bedtime. A little extra precaution is needed when using essential oils in a young child's tub. Unlike adults, who may add essential oils directly to bath water, you must be careful with children. Be sure that no undiluted droplets get rubbed into sensitive eyes. Suggested dilution for a child's bath oil is 1 percent; use one-half to one teaspoon of bath oil for the tub. Bubble baths are another option for the dilution of essential oils for children. Use a pH-balanced shampoo as the soap base.

Part of the elegance of bath oils comes from their containers. Beautiful bottles add glamor to the oils you display in your bathroom or give as gifts. Import stores or mail-order catalogs are a good source of fancy bottles, although we've obtained some of our favorite containers at garage sales and flea markets. Decorate your creations by inserting a few sprigs of dried flowers or dried herbs in clear bottles, or use colored glass containers with a few herbal sprigs tied on the outside with a ribbon.

Floating Aromatic Bath Oil

25 drops essential oil (1/4 teaspoon)
1 ounce vegetable oil

Shake to mix. Use 1 teaspoon per bath. For babies mix 6 drops essential oil to 1 ounce carrier oil, and use 1/2 to 1 teaspoon per bath.

Dispersing Bath Oils

These are scented oils that disperse throughout the bath water. They produce a hint of fragrance without leaving a coating on the skin—perfect for those with oily skin or anyone who finds a floating-oil bath too rich. To get an essential oil to disperse rather than float on top of the water, you need an emulsifier. Commercial bath products use a coconut-oil or chemical-based emulsifier, but egg yolk is an excellent home emulsifier. Another alternative is sulfated castor oil, which is water-soluble. Rather than floating on the surface of the bath, dispersing bath oils blend with the water, making it feel silky.

Hydrous lanolin, another water-soluble substance, makes a richer, more emollient bath oil. Hydrous (meaning "with water") lanolin is easier to work with than sticky, thick anhydrous ("without water") lanolin. Lanolin, derived from sheep's wool, is moisturizing to the skin.

Dispersing Bath Oil

2 ounces sulfated castor oil
1/2 teaspoon essential oil
1/2 teaspoon hydrous lanolin (optional)

If using lanolin, warm it with the castor oil to melt it completely. Add the essential oils after the other oils have cooled. Use 1 teaspoon per bath.

Dispersing Bath Formula

1 egg
10 drops (1/8 teaspoon) essential oil

Separate the egg yolk and discard the white. Mix the essential oil into the yolk, and add the mixture to a full tub. The water will be a bit cloudy, but the essential oil will be distributed evenly.

Aromatic Bath Vinegar

Another variation on the aromatic bath oils are aromatic vinegars, well-suited for oily skin, fungal skin infections, or for anyone sensitive to the alkalinizing effects of soap on their skin. Any type of vinegar will do, but for an attractive display in your bathroom, use red-wine vinegar—which imparts a beautiful color—

and, of course, put it in a clear bottle. Instructions for making herbal vinegars are provided in the appendix to this book.

For dramatic flair, make a vinegar-and-oil dressing. (Body salad, anyone?) Fill the bottle with equal parts bath vinegar and bath oil, and you will have a two-layered bath dressing. The only trick is to make sure that the scents of the bath oil and the vinegar blend pleasantly. Use your imagination to add contrast between the different shades of vegetable oils and vinegars. Keep it in a fancy bottle and shake well before using.

Aromatic Bath Vinegar

25 drops (1/4 teaspoon) essential oil
4 ounces vinegar

Combine ingredients. Let the essential oil sit in the vinegar for a week, shaking the bottle every day. Use 2 tablespoons per bath.

Two-Layered Bath Oil

2 ounces prepared bath oil
2 ounces prepared bath vinegar

Combine and shake well before using.

Aromatic Bath Salts

Bath salts are a luxurious addition to your bath water. They are simple to make, and are always a welcome and exotic gift. They make the water feel silky, remove body oils and perspiration, soften the skin, relax the muscles and soak away the stresses of the day.

Most water in the United States is naturally "hard" because of the calcium and magnesium it contains. Hard water presents no problem until you use it for washing. Then the minerals in the water chemically combine with the free alkali in soap to form an insoluble compound that bears the unattractive name "soap scum," also known as "bathtub ring." Having nowhere else to go, this compound deposits itself in a fine film on skin and hair, leaving them dull and rough.

One solution is to add sodium salts that react with hard minerals to soften water. This makes the water feel silky and smooth, helping soap work better by creating more suds and preventing it from leaving a film residue. An example of this is the addition of washing soda to laundry to prevent hard water from making clothes stiff.

Bath salts are made from very simple ingredients. Any sodium salt will work, but one of the gentlest is common table salt, sodium chloride. Other sodium salts include baking soda, which absorbs odors and relieves itching, and borax. Many companies that make commercial bath salts list these together as "mixed salts," but it is possible to make fine bath salts using just table salt.

For fancy bath salts, the addition of ground seaweed (if you don't mind the smell) or clay will increase the mineral content and make your creation seem more like a treatment at a mineral spa. Using sea salt also contributes tiny amounts of minerals to the bath.

Epsom salts are another type of bath salt, but it is magnesium sulfate and therefore not a water softener. In fact, it is a water hardener, but works much better than other salts to soothe sore muscles, sprains and stiff bodies in general. All salts, especially magnesium, are dehydrating, so use them sparingly if you have dry skin.

Aromatic Bath Salts

1 cup borax
1/2 cup sea salt
1/2 cup baking soda
50 drops essential oil (1/2 teaspoon)

Mix dry ingredients together and add essential oils, mixing well to combine. Use 1/4 to 1/2 cup bath salts per bath. For muscular aches and pains, the addition of 1/2 cup Epsom salts to this recipe is very helpful.

Aromatic Combinations for the Bath

Here are some suggested essential-oil combinations for the recipes given above. Be creative and have fun— the proportions are up to you. Use the blend recipes to make stock bottles of concentrates, which you can later use to create bath oils, bath salts, massage oils and so on.

Relaxing Blend

neroli
marjoram
Roman chamomile
lavender

Stimulating Blend

rosemary
peppermint
lime

Balancing Blend	Aphrodisiac Blend
lavender	sandalwood
geranium	ylang-lang
orange	jasmine

Steam Baths

The Scandinavian steam bath, or sauna, and the Native American sweat lodge both traditionally employ fragrant plants. The herbs are either placed directly on the hot rocks or infused in the water that is poured on the rocks. Cedar leaf and sage are traditionally used for the sweat lodge. Eucalyptus is the most popular essence for steam baths. You can also use essential oils of Himalayan cedar and fir, or place a small amount of the resins frankincense or myrrh directly on the rocks.

Each of these methods encourages sweating, which aids circulation and helps to flush out the system and revitalize the skin. This type of bath ritual was used by many different cultures in the treatment of disease, with some adopting it as part of their spiritual practice.

An Aromatic Bath Experience

Follow these steps to bliss and escape from the world for 40 minutes:

- Light some incense or put a few drops of your favorite essential oil in an electric cooker with a little water, to create a fragrant environment.
- Put on some soothing music.
- Arrange the needed bath materials: thick, scented towel, warm robe, slippers. (You can impart the fragrance of your favorite essential oils to all of your linens by tucking small scented cloths or empty essential-oil bottles into your linen closet.)
- Draw a hot bath.
- Drink a soothing cup of chamomile tea as the tub fills.
- Add half a cup of scented bath salts to the bath water.
- Add one drop of an exotic oil such as rose or jasmine, and swirl to disperse it.
- Light a candle and turn off the lights.
- Step into the bath and relax for 30 minutes with no thoughts of the outside world.
- Emerge, dry off, and dust with a fragrant powder or apply a moisturizing cream to your entire body.
- Wrap up in a warm robe, carry the candle to the bedroom and place a fragrant dream pillow under your bed pillow.
- Slip into bed. Enjoy fragrant dreams and a restful slumber.

Foot or Hand Bath

You may be surprised to learn that herbal and essential-oil foot and hand baths are effective ways of treating problems in other parts of the body. The famous French herbalist Maurice Messegue and aromatherapist Madame Maury did much of their healing work with these baths. Use 5 to 15 drops of essential oil per treatment, depending on how much water is used and essential oils chosen. The soles of the feet and the palms of the hand are much less susceptible to the irritating potential of many essential oils. Water temperature can vary depending on what condition you are treating. Warm or hot water usually feels best, but cold to tepid temperatures are more appropriate for sprains or fevers. Follow your instincts and listen to your body.

AROMATIC BODY POWDERS

Arrowroot, cornstarch and white clay all make good bases for natural aromatic body powders for babies or adults. Commercial powders are usually made with talc (magnesium silicate). In her book *The Consumers Dictionary of Cosmetic Ingredients*, Ruth Winter cites studies identifying talcum powder as a possible carcinogen. A 1972 study by the FDA Office of Product Technology showed that 39 out of 40 talc samples tested contained up to 1 percent asbestos, a proven human carcinogen. Even without asbestos, talc fibers are similar enough in composition to asbestos to pose a potential hazard. Winter also refers to a 1982 article from the journal *Cancer* that links ovarian cancer with talc use. She reports that gynecologist Daniel Cramer found that women who used talcum powder on their genitals and sanitary napkins had more than three times the risk of ovarian cancer, and that the use of talc on latex gloves in surgery contributed to inflammation of the internal organs. Winter further states, "Talcum powder has been reported to cause coughing, vomiting or even pneumonia when it is used carelessly and inhaled by babies."

The addition of finely powdered herbs to your cornstarch- or arrowroot-based body powder can be an added bonus. To blend the essential oils into the powder evenly, put everything through a sieve, mix well and let the mixture sit a few days so that the scents can mellow and evenly permeate the powder. When using any powder, avoid creating a cloud of dust that could be inhaled, especially by babies.

Aromatic Baby Powder

1/4 cup arrowroot
1/4 cup cornstarch
1-2 tablespoons fine white clay
1 teaspoon goldenseal root or myrrh powder
(both are optional, for diaper rash)
3 drops each lavender, Roman chamomile and neroli

Lavender Sunrise Body Powder

1/2 cup powder base
2 tablespoons finely ground and sifted dried lavender flowers
3 drops lavender oil
5 drops rose oil
5 drops orange oil

Men's Powder

1/2 cup powder base
2 tablespoons fine sandalwood powder
5 drops sandalwood oil
3 drops jasmine oil
3 drops lime oil

"Ooh! Ah!" Foot Powder

1/2 cup powder base
5 drops geranium oil
5 drops lavender oil
1 drop cinnamon oil
3 drops rosemary oil

AROMATIC HAIR CARE

There is nothing more radiant than beautiful, shiny, vibrant hair. Short or long, straight or curly, dark or light, hair is truly our crowning glory. It reflects our self-image, and when our mood or lifestyle changes we often change our hair style accordingly. But no matter what the current fashion, clean, healthy hair is always in style. With the help of nature's healing plants, keeping your hair beautiful is easy and fun. Whether it is dry, normal or oily, all hair can benefit from applications of essential oils and herbs.

Hormonal fluctuations, diet, lifestyle and stress play a role in the appearance and health of the hair. The ravages of modern life—including pollution, harsh detergents, chlorine, permanents, blow drying and excessive sun exposure—are just a few of the things that can have an adverse impact on the vitality of your hair. The obvious advice is to correct poor dietary and lifestyle habits, treat your hair with gentle, loving care, and use high-quality natural hair-care products.

For hundreds of years, women have used hair rinses made of vinegar for their softening, pH-balancing effects. Acid shampoos and vinegar alter the electrical charge of the hair, reducing its tendency to become "flyaway." They also cut through soap scum, removing any detergent residues, leaving hair shiny and soft.

"Normal" Hair

If you consider your hair "normal," what you currently use on it is probably fine, but check the label for the pH, as well as for harmful or artificial ingredients. Lavender and rosemary are two good essential oils for normal hair. To apply them, gently comb out wet hair with a wide-toothed comb, working from the ends to the scalp. When the hair is completely dry, put one drop of rosemary essential oil on your palm, rub it into your natural-bristle brush, and brush the hair, again from the ends to the scalp. This helps detangle your hair and makes it smooth, shiny and silky. Too much essential oil can be drying to the hair, so be careful not to overdo it.

Dry Hair

Dry hair and a dry scalp go hand in hand, meaning if you have one you probably have both. When hair becomes dry, the keratin protein it contains turns brittle. Without adequate sebum production by the scalp to protect hair's moisture, it is vulnerable to split ends and can appear unmanageable as well as produce flakes. Drink plenty of water and take a look at your diet to make sure you are getting a sufficient supply of essential fatty acids. A supplement of evening primrose oil or some other oil that contains GLA (gamma-linoleic acid), such as flaxseed oil, is often helpful. Protect dry hair when exposed to drying conditions such as sailing, biking or spending a day at the beach. Dry hair is especially vulnerable to any chemical treatments, from perms and dyes to swimming pool chlorine, which strips away its natural oils.

Avoid daily shampooing, and use mild shampoos containing fatty acids and moisturizers. Unfortunately, protein-rich shampoos cannot feed the hair directly, because the hair shaft is no longer alive. However, a protein film will coat dry hair, allowing it to reflect light and appear shiny. The hair will seem thicker and smoother without a "flyaway" look, at least until the protein coat wears off. High-protein herbs such as comfrey create similar effects. Herbal shampoos smell good, but simply do not remain on the hair long enough to do much good.

Herbal hair conditioners hold more promise, but are best left on at least a few minutes before rinsing. Conditioning herbs for dry hair include calendula, chamomile, lavender, rosemary, sandalwood and burdock root. Hot-oil treatments are specific for dry hair, dry scalp and dandruff. They are simple to prepare, but can be a little messy to apply. Oily hairdressings will help give damaged hair some shine, but they will not always restore its flexibility and bounce. A small amount of sandalwood oil rubbed between your palms and applied to the dry ends of your hair is helpful and leaves a wonderful fragrance that lasts for hours.

Oily Hair

Oily hair is caused by the same condition responsible for oily skin: excess sebum production. Oil comes from the scalp, so the hair is much oilier near the roots than at the tips. Too much oil in the hair makes it look dull, heavy and lifeless. However, the right amount of oil makes the hair look shiny, because it fills in minute abrasions on the surface of the hair shaft. Hormonal changes affect the amount of oil the scalp produces, and diet, as always, may also be a factor.

To remove excess sebum and keep oily hair bright requires frequent washing with a mild shampoo. Harsh detergents can overdry the hair, prompting the sebaceous glands to manufacture more oil. Avoid protein and balsam shampoos because these tend to increase oiliness, make the hair heavy and attract dirt. Seaweed in conditioners may improve matters. Brush oily hair thoroughly before washing.

Essential oils of cedarwood, lemon, lemongrass or sage in your conditioner all discourage oil production by the scalp, as does diluted lemon juice. Adding one drop of patchouli essential oil to your daily dose of shampoo also helps reduce sebum production. Vinegar hair rinses discourage dandruff and keep oily hair in check. If you are concerned about smelling like pickles afterwards, don't worry—the odor of vinegar dissipates within an hour or so. You may also find an herbal rinse of sage tea helpful for reducing dandruff and excess oil.

Shampoo

A good shampoo will clean the hair without stripping away the hair's natural oil, abrading the hair cuticle (resulting in "frizz") or irritating the eyes. Most shampoos are made with sodium lauryl sulfate, a potentially irritating detergent that dramatically increases suds production (something most people expect from a shampoo) in both hard and soft water. Some cosmetic chemists feel that, compared to other cleansing agents, shampoos containing ammonium lauryl sulfate are less irritating. Many shampoos use a base derived from coconut and other nut oils but, surprisingly, some coconut-based products tend to irritate sensitive skin. Baby shampoos are usually mild and pH balanced, and they are often made from olive and soy oil. One place to look for mild shampoos is at a professional hair salon, but check the ingredient labels.

Many books about natural cosmetics give recipes for making herbal shampoos. Most of these are combinations of herb tea and castile soap flakes. We haven't been satisfied with their results because castile soap is very alkaline and leaves the hair feeling stiff and looking dull. There is now a pH-balanced castile soap, although they have merely added vinegar to adjust the pH. Test your brand with nitrizine paper to make sure it has a balanced pH of about 5.

We have seen "European aromatherapy" shampoos that sell for exorbitant prices, but contain nothing more than detergents to clean, vinegar to balance the pH, salt to thicken and essential oils to scent. You can easily and inexpensively make your own formula by mixing equal parts strong herb tea and your chosen shampoo base with a few drops of esssential oil. We like to use a gentle, nondetergent, unscented shampoo as a base. Making small batches (4 ounces) will ensure freshness. Try different combinations of herbs and essential oils to suit your hair type, or simply add two or three drops of essential oil per application to your favorite store-bought shampoo. Your homemade herbal shampoo can also double as a body wash, providing the shampoo base you use is very mild.

Herbal Shampoo

2 ounces unscented shampoo base
2 ounces strong herb tea
30 drops (1/4 teaspoon) essential oil
1/2 ounce vinegar (optional)

Add the strained, cooled tea to the shampoo base. Add the essential oils and shake well before use.

Herbal Hair Rinse

3-5 drops essential oil
1 pint water or herb tea
1 tablespoon vinegar or lemon juice

Shake well, and pour over the scalp and hair after shampooing. Leave on for several minutes and rinse. Refrigerate any leftover rinse.

Aromatic Hair Treatments

Scalp Treatment

This recipe can be used to treat dandruff and falling hair, or to stimulate hair growth, depending on the essential oils you choose.

30 drops (1/4 teaspoon) essential oil
2 ounces carrier (witch hazel, aloe juice, jojoba oil, or neem oil)

Apply to scalp, massage in and cover. Leave it on for one to two hours and shampoo out.

Herbs for Hair Care

Dry	orange peel, calendula, comfrey root
Oily	sage, lemongrass, burdock, lemon peel
Dandruff	burdock, sage, willow bark
Hair loss	nettle, peppermint
All types	lavender, chamomile, rosemary, rose

Essential Oils for Hair Care

Dry	sandalwood, palmarosa, rosewood
Oily	lemongrass, patchouli, clary sage, cypress, cedarwood
Dandruff	sage, geranium, juniper, cedarwood, tea tree
Hair loss	basil, cedarwood, ylang-ylang, peppermint
All types	lavender, Roman chamomile, rosemary, carrot seed

Lice Treatment

Always do a patch test before using this preparation, especially on children. Some people will be sensitive to a solution as strong as this one. Take extra care to keep it out of the eyes and remove at the first sign of any irritation. To thoroughly eliminate lice and hatching eggs, repeat the treatment three times at three-day intervals.

20 drops eucalyptus
10 drops rosemary
10 drops juniper
20 drops lavender
10 drops geranium
5 drops lemon
4 ounces carrier oil

Mix ingredients, apply to dry hair and cover with a plastic bag or a shower cap. Wrap the head in a towel to help keep the vapors from irritating the eyes. Leave the oil on for one to two hours. When you are ready to wash it out, apply shampoo directly to the hair without wetting the hair first; this will help cut the oil. Work the shampoo into the hair well, rinse with water and shampoo again. The final rinse water should contain a few drops of lavender essential oil to further discourage critters. If you are missing any ingredient, substitute tea tree.

Baldness Treatment

Every once in a while, yet another magic formula for reversing baldness is advertised, but so far there is no wonder cure. This harmless but distressful problem mostly afflicts men; more than half of North American men lose their locks to some degree. Thinning usually starts at the temples, and eventually the front hair line and the crown of the head begin to thin. Once the hair is gone, there is little chance that it will return.

There are, however, methods of keeping the remaining hair healthy and on the head as long as possible. In most cases, even if these treatments do not increase hair growth, they can help by slowing further hair loss.

Better than any secret formula, the most effective way to keep hair roots healthy is to stimulate circulation with a scalp-massage formula containing jojoba oil, vitamin E and essential oils that improve circulation, such as rosemary. Aloe vera is said to promote hair growth; some studies back such claims, but others report mixed results. Hair conditioners containing balsams don't actually foster hair growth, but do make the remaining hair seem thicker.

Hair-Growth Formula

50 drops (1/2 teaspoon) rosemary essential oil
1/2 cup aloe-vera gel
1 tablespoon apple-cider vinegar
1 tablespoon wheat-germ or jojoba oil

Shake well and massage into scalp for 10 minutes nightly.

AN AROMATIC MISCELLANY

Nail Care

Neglected, chewed or abused nails just don't get the attention they deserve. Gentle shaping, moisturizing and buffing encourage healthy growth and strengthen the nails. Brittle nails that crack easily indicate possible dietary problems: Are you getting sufficient calcium/magnesium, protein and silica? Detergents, nail polish, glue for artificial fingernails, formaldehyde-based nail hardeners and household chemicals are just a few of the substances that can be tough on fingernails. It is not unusual to develop nail fungus under artificial fingernails.

Herbal-tea soaks or herb-infused oil treatments of comfrey, oat straw and horsetail can strengthen nails and cuticles. Better yet, try combining herbal and essential-oil treatments. Drinking oat straw, nettle and horsetail tea daily can improve your nails (and hair) from the inside out, because these herbs are high in silica and other minerals important for nail growth.

Antifungal Nail Oil

5 drops tea-tree essential oil
1 drop cinnamon-bark essential oil
1/2 ounce neem oil (or calendula-infused oil)

Apply around and under the nail two or three times per day. Tea-tree oil by itself may be used neat if you don't mind the smell, but be careful not to rub it in your eyes.

Aromatic Conditioning Nail Soak

2 drops each lavender, bay laurel and sandalwood essential oils
1/2 ounce jojoba or neem oil

This is great for dry or torn cuticles. Soak nails in the mixture for 10 minutes. Buff to stimulate circulation and bring out a healthy shine.

Natural Deodorant

Sweat is sterile until it comes into contact with airborne bacteria; then by-products created by the interactions break down the bacteria, producing underarm odor. Our culture tends to regard a person's natural scent with some disdain, so antiperspirants are popular. They are made with potentially toxic aluminum compounds that have recently caused some major health concerns. The underarm area is especially sensitive and is notorious for its susceptibility to irritation and rash, and blocking the sweat glands may also be detrimental. We do know that once the effects of an antiperspirant wears off, the underarm sweat glands increase their production of perspiration to make up for the difference. Even the simplest deodorants are often loaded with questionable ingredients and synthetic fragrances. Natural deodorants offer the concerned consumer an alternative. The most important action of any deodorant is to kill bacteria, and natural brands do so with essential oils. Coriander essential oil has been found effective in inhibiting underarm bacterial growth and is used in some natural deodorant products. Roman chamomile oil is also used in a number of natural deodorants, and its anti-inflammatory action is helpful for those with sensitive skin.

If you want a completely pure natural deodorant, why not make one yourself? Some people who don't perspire much find that a simple aromatic body powder will do, but many need a liquid that can be sprayed or sponged on.

Underarm Deodorant

15 drops rosewood oil
5 drops cypress oil
5 drops sage oil
5 drops coriander or lavender oil
2 ounces aloe-vera juice or witch hazel
1 tablespoon alcohol
4 drops grapefruit-seed extract

Combine all ingredients in a spray bottle. Shake well before every application.

Lip Care

Nothing is more sensuous than full, moist lips. Protect them from drying wind and cold conditions by using soothing lip balm, and keep them moist by drinking plenty of water. This recipe will heal chapped lips and keep them kissable.

Lip Balm

1/4 cup herb-infused oil (calendula, chamomile, lavender for healing, or alkanet for red color)
1/4 ounce beeswax, shaved
10-20 (about 1/8 teaspoon) drops essential oil

Follow the directions for making salves in the "Guidelines for Use" chapter. You can alter this formula by choosing different vegetable oils and essential oils. Some suggestions for flavoring lip balms are tangerine, anise, peppermint, neroli and rose essential oils.

9

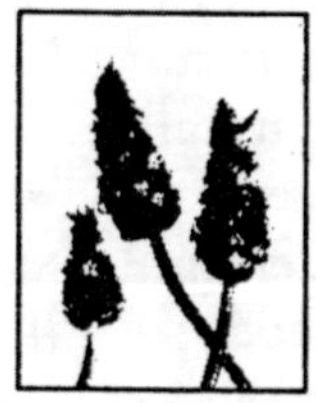

Facial Care

Nature must have designed aromatherapy especially for skin care, because it offers such a complete health and beauty package. Throughout history, aromatherapy has cleared complexions, softened hands and made hair silky for the world's most beautiful women. These beauties knew the secrets nature holds in her botanical collection. The formulas they passed down to us reveal that plants—especially those containing essential oils—were the key ingredients in their cosmetics.

Modern skin-care products are sold with slick advertising and dazzling packages. Although the array of products may feel, smell and look different, they are quite similar. Most products follow a basic formula. Behind fancy labels claiming "new" or "improved" ingredients, they consist of mineral oil and water held together with synthetic waxes and emulsifiers, and scented with artificial fragrances. Myriad "new" chemical ingredients are also added to make the products look and feel more appealing.

Appealing, that is, until you begin to read the fine print on the labels. Today's more sophisticated cosmetic labels often include names that require a chemical dictionary to comprehend. Reconstructed lanolin and other "chemically altered" emulsifiers and stabilizers help assure that the ingredients don't separate no matter how much heat, cold or shaking they endure during the long journey from manufacturing plant to your home. The result is a seminatural or semisynthetic product, depending on which way you want to look at it.

The word *cosmetic* comes from the Greek word *kosmos,* meaning "order" or "harmony." We believe in turning to nature for the most harmonizing ingredients. Many cosmetic firms now add botanical derivatives as "active" ingredients to cash in on the trend toward natural ingredients, but a few companies truly concerned about skin care are making an effort to produce totally natural products. Read labels carefully when choosing skin-care products.

If you have the time, you too can make aromatherapy body-care products—for only a fraction of what you pay in the store. To inspire your creations, we've included our favorite recipes. Instructions for treating your specific skin type are explained below. First, we'll take a close look at skin care to help you make informed decisions about the products you buy and make.

The most important element for the skin is water. Healthy skin is 50-75 percent water, which keeps skin cells soft and supple, decreasing flakiness, dryness and wrinkles. Unfortunately, the skin constantly loses water through sweat and evaporation. To help retain this precious commodity, sebaceous glands (tiny coiled structures that lie next to hair follicles) secrete an oil called *sebum,* which coats the skin. Water-attracting compounds, collectively called "natural moisturizing factors" (NMFs), also help to retain water.

Another important factor to consider is the skin's acid-alkaline balance. Healthy skin is slightly acid, pH

4.5 to 5.5. (The pH scale goes from acid to alkaline, 0 to 14, 7 being "neutral.") Called the "acid mantle," this protective barrier keeps out harmful bacteria and other potential pathogens. You can test the pH of any cosmetic product with nitrazine paper in the 4.5 to 7.5 range, available from your local pharmacy.

BEAUTY TECHNIQUES

Beauty isn't just skin deep—it also reflects your inner health. To maintain a radiant complexion from the inside out and assist the cells in all of their metabolic functions, eat a balanced diet and get plenty of rest and exercise to improve circulation. Encourage natural collagen production by taking vitamin C, including the entire complex of rutin, bioflavonoids and hesperidin. (Two of the most destructive influences on collagen are sun exposure and cigarette smoking.) Choose skin products that are in the same pH range as skin. Keep skin moisturized by drinking plenty of water. Although scientific studies don't correlate water consumption with skin hydration, estheticians urge their clients to drink six to eight glasses each day to avoid skin dryness.

A good rule of thumb (though maybe a bit purist) concerning product ingredients is to never put anything on your face that you couldn't put in your mouth. Though all of our suggestions for product ingredients are natural, some highly sensitive individuals may have allergies to a few of them. It's a good idea to test any suspected ingredients for sensitivities. See the safety precautions in the "Guidelines" chapter, and test as you would for an essential oil.

One of the very best things you can do to promote a glowing complexion is an aromatherapy facial treatment. The basic techniques are cleansing, steaming, exfoliation, mask application, toning and moisturizing. How you employ these methods, as well as your choice of essential oils and herbs, should be determined by your skin type. We describe all the facial techniques in this chapter, then give guidelines on how to custom-design these methods for your own skin type.

Cleansers

Beware of many of the skin-cleansing products on the market. Like soap, many are alkaline so they can clean and penetrate skin better. This translates to harshness on your skin as they strip away the natural protective acid mantle, leaving it vulnerable to bacteria and encouraging the production of rough callous cells in self-defense. Healthy skin produces lactic acid and eventually regains its acid mantle, but this is not an easy task for all skin types. Dry skin is especially susceptible to problems with alkaline cleansers. The result is extreme dryness with sallow appearance and rough texture.

Most bar soaps are alkaline, and many are made with synthetic or partially synthetic ingredients. Sodium lauryl sulfate is the basis of most liquid facial and body soaps, as well as shampoos. Even if pH-balanced and filled with natural ingredients, such soaps can still be harsh on sensitive skin. The most critical review of sodium lauryl sulfate comes from chemist and natural-cosmetics manufacturer Kurt Schnaubelt, who notes: "Sodium lauryl sulfate and related detergents [may] cause eye irritations, skin rashes, hair loss, scalp scurf similar to dandruff and allergic reactions. According to a report released by the FDA in 1978, it can combine with other chemicals [such as emulsifiers, TEA and DEA] to create the cancer-causing N-nitrosamines." Alternatives do exist, such as potassium coco protein and glycin cleansers, which are difficult but not impossible to find. (See "Resources.") Ground oatmeal is good for washing the face, and in the section of this chapter on cleansers we present a recipe for a homemade cleanser using aloe vera and grapefruit-seed extract.

Before cleansing, remove makeup with homemade cream or vegetable oil. Gently wash your face with warm water, using the cleanser most appropriate for your complexion type, and pat dry.

Steaming

Steaming is an excellent way to moisturize the skin and increase circulation. It will help clean the skin, and leave your face looking youthful and vibrant. Steaming won't remove dirt and grime, but will help soften sebum and unclog pores. Steaming can be done once a week on most skin types—except for couperose (see "Skin Types" below), extremely delicate or extremely dry skin that may be irritated by heat.

Steam carries volatile oils directly to the face, so essential oils or fragrant herbs can be added to the steam water. Nonfragrant herbs, such as comfrey or plantain, are healing when applied to the skin, but are useless in steam because they contain no essential oil. In preparing a "facial sauna," brew a strong infusion (tea) using fragrant herbs with boiling water, or by adding a few drops of essential oil to plain steaming water. Set up the pan in a location where you can comfortably sit next to it. Lay a towel over the back of your head, put your face over the steam, and secure the ends of the towel around the pan to capture all the steam, creating a miniature sauna. Keep your eyes closed so that the essential-oil-filled steam will not irritate them, and keep your face about 12 inches from the steam source. Enjoy the relaxing warmth for a minute or so, then remove your head, taking a few breaths of fresh air if needed. Go back under the towel and repeat a few times. We recommend that you steam for no longer than 5 or 10 minutes, depending on your skin type. The water or tea from the steam can be saved for your final rinse water. (Just make sure it has cooled sufficiently.)

If you are in a hurry or traveling and need a quick steam method, place two herbal tea bags (such as chamomile or mint) in a cup and pour boiling water over them. Then steam your face over the cup of fragrant vapors.

Exfoliates

Exfoliation is the removal of dead skin cells from the epidermis, the skin's outer layer. Done properly, this brings young, fresh skin to the surface and stimulates cell growth in the lower layers. Exfoliation also gives the impression of erasing wrinkles, because it removes cell buildup on the skin that makes lines appear deeper. Most skin types benefit from exfoliation, but be especially gentle with sensitive, thin or couperose skin. If overdone, exfoliation can be irritating as it exposes underlying skin before it is ready to face the world. Do not exfoliate too often, and avoid chemical exfoliants such as those used in some beauty salons.

Some exfoliants, such as cornmeal, work by gentle abrasion, whereas others, such as papaya, pineapple and ginger, have an enzymatic action on the skin. Among the newest cosmetic ingredients are alpha-hydroxy acids (AHAs), which encourage exfoliation by loosening the tight bond that holds surface skin together. Fine lines become smoother, skin texture becomes softer, spotty skin pigmentation becomes more even and, because AHAs are antibacterial, acne problems improve. In addition, the naturally high acidity in AHAs restores the acid mantle of the skin. (Dermatologists even use highly concentrated solutions to remove scar tissue.) Since AHAs are also good moisturizers, they provide a very gentle way to exfoliate sensitive skin. AHAs are common in many cosmetic products today, including cleansers, toners, masks and moisturizers. For use as a product ingredient, you can buy AHAs in liquid form (such as a prepared toner, available at most natural-food stores), so it can be easily added to your homemade cosmetics.

The use of alpha-hydroxy acids is not really a new idea; women have been putting them on their faces for centuries. Nature offers a variety: glycolic acid is found in certain fruits and sugar, lactic acid in yogurt and sour milk, acetic acid in vinegar, malic acid in apples, citric acid in citrus fruits, tartaric acid in wine. Cleopatra bathed in milk, 18th-century European women splashed wine on their faces, and the practice of applying yogurt, sour milk or fruit to the face is an ancient beauty secret. (Try starting your day with a yogurt-and-fruit smoothy for breakfast, then spread some of it on your face!)

Dermatologist Ruey J. Yu of Temple University in Philadelphia has been studying the effects of alpha-hydroxy acids on skin since the early 1980s. He feels that one reason physical exercise may be so good for the skin is that sweat contains lactic acid and moisturizes the skin. The only problem is that most people shower with soap shortly after exercising. The soap removes the lactic acid and dries the skin.

Choose an exfoliant or scrub appropriate for your skin type. Apply in gentle, circular movements. Some exfoliants double as cleansers, masks or toners.

Masks

Masks can absorb, moisturize, feed or remineralize the skin. Many good masks can easily be made at home for pennies. Choose ingredients suitable for your skin type. Several clays may be used as a base: white and green clays are for any skin type; red or yellow clays are very absorptive for oily skin; and gentle blue clay is for sensitive or couperose skin. The colors are natural and reflect the minerals found in the clay.

Clay is the most drying of the masks, but this can be adjusted with other ingredients. Honey or foods naturally high in oil (such as avocado or cream) are least drying. Eggs, fresh fruits and vegetables, oats, cream of wheat, yogurt and nutritional yeast are just a few of the other possibilities for mask ingredients. Fruits and herbs containing skin-softening enzymes act as exfoliants and may be incorporated into masks. These can also be combined with other skin-care products to soften and smooth rough skin. Essential oils or ground herbs can be added to increase the skin-healing properties of the mask.

To make a mask, mash the ingredients into a thick paste, adding hydrosols, herb tea or aloe to moisten the dry ingredients. (We suggest oats or clay.) Apply to the face in an even layer. Avoid sensitive areas around the eyes and the edges of the mouth. Following this step, lie down and relax. Feel the mask working, and visualize yourself with radiant skin.

Facial masks can be left on from 5 to 20 minutes, as long as the mask remains comfortable. This varies with skin type and mask ingredients, but don't allow the mask to dry or pull so much that it becomes irritating. Wash the mask off with warm water and gently pat the skin dry.

Toners

Toners can do wonders for the complexion. They increase circulation, giving your face a healthful glow, improve skin tone, and reduce wrinkles and enlarged pores—at least temporarily. Toners are often astringent, drawing water from underlying skin levels to the surface. This extra water makes the skin puff up slightly, so lines and pores seem smaller. The illusion, unfortunately, has a "Cinderella" effect—in a few hours, the magic wears off as the water is reabsorbed and evaporates. Many commercial toners plump the skin with irritating ingredients that cause a slight inflammation, thus diminishing lines. Some are high in alcohol to help remove the mineral oil used in most cleansers.

Toners can also serve as moisturizers and offer a good alternative to oil-based moisturizers for those with very oily or problem skin. AHAs or aloe vera are excellent for these skin types. They are also suitable for normal to dry complexions when combined with a small amount of oil or glycerin. They can help heal psoriasis, eczema, blemishes, and infections that result from either acne or dry skin. Some individuals are sensitive to aloe vera (or the additives in commercial brands), so test it first somewhere other than the face. Because of their acidic nature, AHAs can cause a slight burning, depending on the strength. Diluting them will alleviate the problem, but they won't be as "active."

Facial toners can be made with plain apple cider, wine or other vinegars. Avoid white vinegar derived from petroleum. (White corn vinegar is fine.) Cosmetic vinegars can be infused with herbs to boost their healing properties. Vinegars were the rage for centuries, but they lost their popularity with the arrival of modern cosmetics that didn't carry that distinctive odor. However, don't let the smell deter you from using vinegar—it lingers only for a short while. Vinegar softens skin, restores the acid mantle, relieves itching, and destroys fungus and yeast (such as candida). A vinegar-based toner used with a moisturizer is excellent for normal to dry skin; when used alone, it has a slight drying effect on oily skin. All toners made with vinegar must be diluted in water, aloe or hydrosol. Use a maximum of one tablespoon vinegar per one-half cup water, or less vinegar for sensitive skin.

Witch hazel from any drugstore can be used as a toner. When you infuse the witch hazel with herbs (just as you would when making an herb-infused vinegar—see "Guidelines"), the 20-percent alcohol content helps extract important plant constituents that are beneficial for the skin. It is also possible to get an aromatic hydrosol of witch hazel without alcohol, but in the recipes in this chapter we are referring to the drugstore type. (In the 15th and 16th centuries, facial toners made with alcohol doubled as potable cordials, sipped by women in the privacy of their dressing rooms!) Alcohol-based toners are acceptable for problem and oily skin and for dabbing on blemishes, but they are not the best choice for dry, delicate or mature skin.

Toner ingredients can be combined. For example, blend aloe-vera juice with a vinegar that has been infused with herbs and add essential oils. Or mix hydrosols with AHAs. Toners can be misted or splashed on, or applied with cotton pads. Toners applied with cotton remove oil and dirt, making adequate cleansers if you're traveling or camping.

Aromatic Hydrosols

Aromatic hydrosols (also known as hydrolats) are so effective as toners, and for skin care in general, that we have given them their own section. An aromatic hydrosol produced during essential-oil distillation can be a valuable addition to your beauty regimen. Hydrosols are impregnated with water-soluble (hydrophilic) compounds that are not present in essential oils. For example, soothing, anti-inflammatory carboxylic acids are found almost exclusively in hydrosols. Mildly astringent yet nondrying, they are ideal for severe cases of psoriasis or highly sensitive skin, or for any case where essential oils might be too strong. Most hydrosols are good to use on normal and oily complexions (or on acne skin), and many are suitable for dry skin. All of them counteract the drying effects encountered on long airplane flights, as well as in air-conditioned rooms and cars. The benefits are especially noticeable when used daily.

Aromatic hydrosols can be used alone as toners, or added to other toner ingredients, such as aloe vera. They are wonderful in masks and lotions. A wide range of pure aromatic hydrosols generally are not available at retail outlets, but they can be purchased by mail order.

Here are examples of hydrosols with cosmetic applications:

German chamomile—for sensitive skin and inflammation.

Helichrysum—rejuvenates damaged or mature skin, heals and soothes inflamed skin conditions.

Lavender—balances all skin types. Soothes sunburns, irritations, psoriasis and eczema.

Lemon verbena—lemon-scented and mildly astringent for oily skin; the odor is light, clean and refreshing.

Melissa—very gentle on sensitive skin.

Myrtle—soothing and gentle, myrtle is also used as an eyewash for irritations and allergic reactions.

Orange blossom—good for couperose, dry or sensitive skin; the delicate fragrance soothes and calms.

Rose—mildly astringent for couperose skin, but suitable for all skin types; good on cotton pads for irritated eyes.

Rosemary—for sluggish, sallow, devitalized skin that needs stimulation and regeneration.

Witch Hazel—astringent for oily or couperose skin, and good as an aftershave tonic.

Yarrow—mildly scented antiseptic, and astringent for problem or oily skin.

Fragrant Waters

Fragrant waters are made by adding essential oils to distilled water. We call them "fragrant waters" to distinguish them from true aromatic hydrosols. They are inexpensive but less effective as moisturizing agents, because they don't contain the same hydrophilic compounds as hydrosols. Adding aloe-vera juice to fragrant waters can boost the moisturizing properties if you want to use them as toners or as cosmetic body mists.

Fragrant waters have many uses, depending on the essential oils you choose. Spray or splash on fragrant water after your daily shower to cool down on a hot day, or whenever you are in the mood for instant aromatherapy. We use them to freshen our faces—and attitudes—on long car trips. Fragrant waters are easy to make, and allow the application of diluted essential oils to your skin without the use of vegetable oil.

Moisturizers

Oil alone is no solution to dry skin; although it adds a silky texture to skin-care products and reduces water loss, no amount of oil by itself can moisturize the skin. However, oil does provide a protective barrier that prevents water from evaporating from the skin's surface, and it smooths rough, scaly skin cells. Water on its own, meanwhile, evaporates quickly from the surface of the skin, causing further dryness. The perfect skin solution is a cream or lotion that brings together the best of both worlds—water to keep skin youthful, fresh and plump, oil to hold back water evaporation.

Facial creams generally consist of 40-60 percent oil and are suitable for dry-skin problems. Heavy, rich creams with more oil offer greater protection, but are greasier and reserved, usually, for the sensitive skin around the eyes that has no oil glands. Standard lotions made with 50-90 percent water are absorbed and spread more easily than creams, making them well suited for normal to oily skin, or as body or massage lotions.

Liposomes are a popular addition to many cosmetics, especially moisturizers, which contain phospholipids (oils) similar to those found in the skin. They bond to the keratin protein produced by the epidermis (the skin's outer layer), creating a lipophilic film that reduces water loss in the deeper layers of the skin. They also act as carriers to deliver other beneficial substances to the deepest layers of the skin, where new cells are formed. In fact, both liposomes and essential oils are so efficient at permeating the skin you need to be careful about what you combine with them. Do not use them with cosmetics containing artificial ingredients, and wait at least 15 minutes after using them before applying foundation or sunscreen.

Liposomes come as a thin emulsion, much like a watery lotion, and are derived from animal or plant sources. (We recommend the vegetable source derived from soybeans.) They can be used undiluted on the skin, but this is very expensive. A 10-percent solution is sufficient in a lotion or cream recipe—and probably much more than this is added to most commercial cosmetics. Liposomes can be combined with essential oils and are useful for all skin types.

Facial oils made with essential oil diluted to 2-3 percent in a carrier oil offer a simple, easy-to-prepare alternative to making your own creams and lotions. They do not contain the water that creams and lotions provide, but when applied directly after a toner are effective skin treatments. Liposomes can also be added to facial oils, but because the watery liposomes separate from the oil, the mixture should be shaken before use.

Apply moisturizers in a thin layer over the entire face and neck while the skin is still damp with toner to help seal in precious moisture. Don't forget to moisturize ear lobes and neck, right down to the collar bone.

Herbs and Essential Oils for the Skin

A number of essential oils can be used for all skin types. Lavender, geranium, rose, neroli and ylang-ylang are so versatile or balancing that many aromatherapists recommend them for more than one skin type. Essential oils can be incorporated into any step of the facial-care routine.

The diverse actions of some herbs make them appropriate candidates for all skin types. Calendula, papaya, chamomile, comfrey, ginseng, horsetail, roses and lavender are just a few of the plants that benefit all skin types and conditions. Their actions are soothing, anti-inflammatory, healing and nutritive. Gotu kola and echinacea are helpful in strengthening connective tissue and increasing the elasticity of the skin. Herbs can be used as a steam or incorporated into skin-product recipes in the form of teas, tinctures and oils. See your skin-type category (below) for specific oils.

Skin-Care Properties of Essential Oils

Here are just some of the effects of essential oils upon the skin:

- penetrate to the dermal layer of skin where new cells are developing;
- stimulate and regenerate; produce healthy skin cells quickly following sun damage, burns, wrinkles or healing of wounds;
- reduce bacterial and fungal infections, acne and other related skin problems;
- soothe delicate, sensitive, inflamed skin;
- regulate sebaceous secretions, balancing over- or underactive skin;
- promote the release and removal of metabolic waste products;
- contain plant "hormones" that help balance and alleviate hormonally related skin problems;
- affect the mental and emotional state positively, thus alleviating stress-related skin problems.

Home Facial Routine

A facial is a real gift to yourself. Better yet, share the experience with a friend. The routine is simple. After doing it a couple of times, you will feel comfortable enough to alter it according to your own preferences and create your own recipes. A facial is easily completed in 20-40 minutes. If you don't have a spare 30 minutes, do a minifacial by steaming clean skin (or applying a mask), then using a moisturizer.

To begin your facial, put on a blouse with a wide or low neck, and pull your hair away from your face. Now gather your materials. You'll need two soft towels, a facial sponge or washcloth, a pan for heating water, a small mixing bowl for the mask or scrub, and all your facial ingredients. Keep your supplies in a box or basket for convenient access whenever you or a friend want a facial.

The steps and time required as as follows:

1. Cleanse—2 minutes
2. Steam—5 to 10 minutes
3. Exfoliate—3 minutes (with facial scrub)
4. Mask—5 to 20 minutes
5. Tone—1 minute.
6. Moisturize—1 minute

The difference in your complexion after a facial will be quite noticeable. We always make sure to bring a mirror to facial classes so participants can see for themselves how radiant and youthful they look afterward. We have many good stories, but our favorite is about the woman who left an evening facial class and, having nowhere else to take her new complexion, went out for a drink. A handsome young man asked her out, and although she was very flattered, she declined—and never did tell him that she was almost 20 years his senior! We can't always promise results like that, but we're sure you'll find the facial experience enjoyable and the results rewarding.

SKIN TYPES

The eight skin types we will discuss are "normal," dry, oily, combination, problem, couperose, mature and sun-damaged. Observe your complexion carefully and read the descriptions to determine your skin type. If you are unsure of your skin type, you can help diagnose it by testing the oil production of your skin with the following blotting test. Go to bed without applying any facial products. In the morning, before washing or putting anything on your face, pat a few strips of a clean brown paper bag on different areas of your face, especially in the "T zone" of chin, nose and forehead. Normal skin areas will show a small amount of oil, oily skin will leave a definite oil stain, and dry skin won't leave any oil on the paper. Even though the cheeks will probably not show any oil stains, feel them for dryness.

Many people experience symptoms that fall into more than one skin-type category. Custom-design your skin treatments by reading the appropriate sections, then choosing techniques and ingredients to suit you. Expect your skin type to change with your menstrual cycle, age, diet, the season and other environmental factors. Typically, skin is "normal" for children, becomes oily during adolescence and gradually becomes drier as we grow older. Women (especially those who are fair-skinned) tend to have drier skin than men, and dryness increases after age 40. As skin matures, you'll need to gradually adjust the way you care for it.

Poor diet or digestion, a sluggish liver, radical changes in weight, lack of exercise, smoking, alcohol consumption, stress or a generally poor lifestyle all contribute to skin problems. The remedies for these are pretty obvious, and there is only so much you can expect from essential oils and herbs if these factors are not alleviated. The basics of daily skin care are cleansing, toning and moisturizing. The complete facial routine adds steaming, exfoliation and a mask. If you can incorporate this regimen into your life once a week, your skin will thank you with a radiant glow.

"Normal" Skin

Ah, to be blessed with "normal" skin—neither too dry nor too oily, but moist and clear, with even texture, color and pore size. "Normal" skin can usually withstand less attention than other skin types, so count your blessings—but don't neglect your skin! You have a wider choice of ingredients than people with other skin types.

CLEANSER: Cleansing can be done once or twice a day with a pH-balanced cream or homemade cleanser.

STEAMING: Once or twice a week will suffice for "normal" skin.

EXFOLIATION: A gentle oatmeal scrub once a week, or daily use of AHAs, will help maintain "normal" skin.

MASK: Almost any type, from clay to yogurt, is suitable.

TONER: Aloe vera or hydrosols are best.

MOISTURIZER: Use light lotions as needed.

ESSENTIAL OILS: Lavender, rose, geranium and neroli are all good for "normal" skin. Feel free to add the oils mentioned for other skin types if your skin condition fluctuates.

HERBS: Calendula, comfrey, roses and lavender.

Dry Skin

Dry skin typically has a fine texture with no visible pores. It feels tight and dry, especially after washing, and is usually caused by underactive oil glands that do not lubricate the skin adequately. Dehydrated skin, which produces enough oil but does not retain enough moisture, is often mistaken for dry skin. Dry skin tends to be sensitive and is susceptible to premature wrinkling and flaking, which is sometimes due to a lack of keratin. It also tends to be thin due to heredity or a lack of the water that would help "plump" it up. Low hormone production can also contribute to dry skin. Dry skin is particularily vulnerable to environmental factors such as wind, the hot conditions of summer, and winter's chapping cold, all of which suppress oil-gland activity. Escaping the heat of summer by jumping into chlorinated swimming pools, or living in the low humidity produced by air-conditioning, present special problems for people with dry skin.

CLEANSER: Dry skin that is not subjected to makeup, poor air quality or dirt may need cleansing only once a day. Foaming cleansers are too drying for this skin type. Use a water-soluble cleansing cream that does not remove the skin's natural oil, or use a custom-made cleanser. Gently pat the face dry.

STEAMING: A facial steam can benefit dry skin, but don't overexpose the face to high heat. Cool it down by letting some steam escape during the treatment. Make the entire session short, five minutes at the most. And do not steam too often—once every week or two is sufficient.

EXFOLIATION: A gentle herbal scrub is ideal because the rubbing stimulates oil production and exfoliates flaky, dry surface skin. Commercial scrubs often use abrasives such as almond shells, but we prefer the gentle effect of finely ground oatmeal. Make a paste of the oatmeal and gently massage the face for one minute.

MASK: An emollient mask with ingredients such as honey, yogurt, avocado and egg yolks aids dry skin because it simultaneously coaxes water to the skin's surface and moisturizes. Masks that are beneficial but potentially drying, such as oatmeal, should be used sparingly or applied briefly so you don't end up with even drier skin. A light application of a moisturizing cream before the mask application may prevent problems. If you do use clay, add a little oil to the mixture and remove it with warm water before it dries completely.

TONER: Avoid products containing alcohol. Instead, use aloe vera or a moisturizing hydrosol such as rose to increase the skin's water content. Diluted apple-cider vinegar is excellent because it softens skin, restores the acid mantle, and relieves the itchiness and flakiness that often accompanies dryness.

MOISTURIZER: Treat dry skin to rich facial creams, especially those that include liposomes. When you wear a foundation makeup, choose one that contains moisturizers. Dry skin also benefits from products that include a small amount of glycerin, which attracts water.

ESSENTIAL OILS: Essential oils for dry skin are palmarosa, rosemary (chemotype verbenone), carrot seed, rosewood and sandalwood. German chamomile reduces puffiness and inflammation of delicate skin. Both chamomile and lavender soothe and heal irritation that can easily develop as outer layers of dry skin flake off. To balance oil-gland production, use lavender and geranium. Neroli oil promotes cell rejuvenation, and the hydrosol is moisturizing. Small amounts of peppermint or rosemary stimulate oil production and increase circulation.

HERBS: For dry skin, use herbs that heal irritated, injured skin, such as violet flowers, red clover and marshmallow. Rosemary helps stimulate underactive skin. Comfrey leaves soothe and mend damaged skin, and St. John's wort helps heal damaged nerves in the underlying tissue. Elder flowers improve skin tone and texture and soothe dry, chafed skin. These herbs are best used in emollient skin creams. Supplements of GLA (gamma-linoleic acids), such as evening primrose oil, can improve dry skin from the inside.

Oily Skin

Large pores, a thick, coarse texture and overactive oil glands give this skin type its characteristic shine. Excess oil tends to attract dirt that can breed bacteria and infection, clogging pores with dead cells. On the positive side, oiliness protects and lubricates skin as it matures, so that fewer wrinkles develop.

In summer, overexposure to the sun stimulates overactive oil glands into even heavier production. The oil also combines with sweat, making skin feel still oilier. In winter, oil buildup is worsened by bundling up with scarves and hats, and by the tendency to wash your face less often. Nothing you use on your skin should completely eliminate oil production, but many natural ingredients can reduce excessive oil production and accumulation. Restricting dietary fat, especially fried foods, would also be appropriate.

CLEANSER: Cleanse oily skin often—at least twice a day—with neutral pH soap (or cleansing gel) and water to remove excess oil.

STEAMING: Steaming can benefit oily skin by unclogging pores and releasing excess oil. This skin type is usually sturdy and can benefit from once- or twice-weekly steam treatments, but monitor your skin and reduce the number of treatments when sebum production decreases.

EXFOLIATION: Avoid vigorous scrubbing that can stimulate oil production. Instead, use gentle oatmeal with cornmeal or powdered herbs as a mild abrasive.

MASK: Facial masks made with oats or clay effectively draw out and absorb surface skin oils. Clay masks should be rinsed off before they begin to feel tight and itchy. Beaten egg whites make a good astringent mask.

TONER: Aloe vera, hydrosols and witch hazel improve the complexion without adding oil. A slight amount of grain alcohol may be used on very oily skin, but if you dry the skin with too much alcohol, it produces even more oil to compensate. Preferably, make a tincture using witch-hazel extract or vinegar instead of alcohol, then add herbs and essential oils specific for oily skin. Wipe away excess oil throughout the day with cotton pads soaked with toner.

MOISTURIZER: Even oily skin needs some moisturizing. When you provide the skin with a little oil, it will produce less of its own sebum. Make a light lotion or facial oil. If you really object to using oil on the face, use aloe gel with essential oils that balance oil production.

ESSENTIAL OILS: The essential oils basil, eucalyptus, cedarwood, cypress, lemongrass, spike lavender and ylang-ylang help to normalize overactive sebaceous glands. Sage and lemongrass also slow down oil production, as well as subdue overactive sudoriferous (sweat) glands. All of the citruses may be used, but keep in mind their photosensitizing effects.

HERBS: Herbs with astringent and drying properties include yarrow and witch hazel. They can be used in tea form as a final rinse after cleansing, or tinctured into witch-hazel extract or vinegar.

Combination Skin

Combination skin—oily in the "T zone" and dry around the eyes, cheeks and mouth—is the most common skin type. Treat combination skin like two separate faces, using a combination of essential oils and herbs. Read the sections on dry and oily skin, and follow the guidelines.

ESSENTIAL OILS: Geranium, lavender, ylang-ylang and rose are considered "normalizers" and play double-duty by treating both oily and dry skin conditions.

HERBS: Calendula, lavender, rose, chickweed, plantain and marshmallow root.

Problem Skin

Pimples, cysts, blackheads and whiteheads can occur in both dry or oily skin. Oily skin with a fine texture and small pore size is the most likely candidate for problem skin. Besides all the contributing lifestyle factors, sluggish liver function is involved. Acne occurs most often where oil glands predominate—on the face, back and chest. Many dermatologists do not agree, but when researchers at Boston University asked patients what triggered their acne, most said stress. Although stress stimulates production of adrenal hormones in both men and women, female acne patients seem to overproduce the hormone testosterone, the cause of most acne. If your acne is hormone-related, it will generally manifest around the chin and jawline. Acne can also be caused by some pharmaceutical drugs, such as those that treat epilepsy or alter hormone production.

Problem skin may be temporary, especially as it occurs during puberty when hormones rage and cause excess oil production, affecting 80 percent of North American adolescents. However, acne does follow many people into adulthood, particularly if it is hormone-related. Normally, oil travels to the skin surface through hair follicles, but when dead cells and excess oil build up, pores become clogged and the hair canal narrows. The resulting lack of oxygen in the pores encourages bacterial growth, which causes inflammation, infection and pustules that can leave scars or pits in the skin. If pores are repeatedly clogged, they enlarge, changing the texture of the skin. Oil trapped in pores can also turn into blackheads, which turn dark as the oil oxidizes. (This darkening is not caused by dirt, as many people mistakenly believe.)

Acne usually improves in early summer as increased sun exposure provides vitamin D and lightly exfoliates the skin, but it can worsen if the oil-producing glands are stimulated by too much heat and sun.

CLEANSER: Problem skin needs thorough cleansing. Follow our advice for oily skin, and cleanse the face as often as three times daily. Many people with problem skin like foaming cleansers; just be sure to choose one that is pH-balanced. If your problem skin is dry, follow the instructions described in that section.

STEAMING: Steaming acne skin once or twice a week can be helpful, but if pustules open you may need to lightly cleanse, or at least rinse, the skin before continuing your facial.

EXFOLIATION: Scrubbing exfoliants can aggravate acne. AHAs will help exfoliate and can double as a toner. A papaya mask will gently exfoliate.

MASK: An astringent mask on problem skin promotes mild peeling and helps reduce large pores. Clay is useful, especially when moistened with toner and mixed with antibacterial essential oils.

TONER: Diluted cider vinegar has antiseptic properties and helps maintain the skin's acid balance. Aloe vera, with its skin-healing properties and pH of 4.3, is an excellent toner or cosmetic base for oily-skin products. Hydrosols are good antiseptics and can be used for problem skin that is oily or dry.

MOISTURIZER: Use light lotions containing mostly aloe vera to help heal damaged skin.

ESSENTIAL OILS: The antiseptic and drying essential oils are spike lavender, juniper, eucalyptus and sage. Rosemary (chemotype verbenone), tea tree and thyme (chemotype linalol) are suitable for problem skin that is dry. Lavender, neroli and rosemary also stimulate new cell growth. In a study of 124 acne patients, a 5-percent dilution of tea-tree oil in a gel base was effective. Although it was slower-acting than the 5-percent benzyl peroxide lotion typically prescribed, it was better tolerated by the skin. The researchers suggested that a stronger solution of tea tree might be ideal. Because tea tree is generally not irritating, most people have no adverse reactions to a stronger solution. Peppermint and sage are antibacterial agents. Chamomile reduces inflammation and softens the skin. You can do neat (undiluted) spot applications of tea tree, lavender, Eucalyptus dives or spike lavender several times a day on pimples or aggravating cystic acne that never comes to a head. This may eventually result in drying, but can be used for two or three days before it becomes a problem.

HERBS: Many herbs come to the rescue of problem skin. Elder flowers, red clover and licorice help unclog pores while refining, softening and healing the complexion. Strawberry leaves discourage excessive oil production. If you make your own products, add herbal tinctures such as goldenseal and myrrh to fight infection, prevent blemishes and encourage healing.

Problem skin may benefit greatly from liver herbs taken internally. Milk thistle, burdock, yellow dock, turmeric and sarsaparilla are especially important to use in conjunction with aromatherapy treatments. They should be taken daily as teas or tinctures.

Couperose Skin

Couperose describes skin marked with tiny dilated capillaries that are not very noticeable, unless the case is severe, and are found mostly around the nose or on the cheeks. This condition can be found in any skin type, but it is most common with dry, thin, delicate or mature skin. It often afflicts people of Northern European descent, especially blonds, redheads or those with very fair skin. It can also be caused and aggravated by exposure to extreme temperatures, alcohol consumption, smoking, high blood pressure or any harsh treatment of the skin that causes capillaries to break. It is a difficult problem to treat, but improvement will be observed over time if the skin is cared for properly. Helpful measures include exercise to increase circulation, aromatherapy treatments, and vitamins, especially those that increase capillary strength, such as E, B_2 and the C complex (bioflavonoids, hesperidin and rutin).

CLEANSER: Take extra care of couperose skin by using tepid water in daily cleansing with a cream cleanser. Never use a cold-water splash.

STEAMING: Avoid steaming unless you keep the sessions short, and expose your face to only moderate heat by holding it far from the steaming pot.

EXFOLIATION: Take extra care when exfoliating couperose skin. Use gentle AHAs such as yogurt or apply a papaya mask, but avoid scrubs, which increase surface circulation and encourage broken capillaries in such sensitive skin.

MASK: Fruit, yogurt or honey masks are the most gentle for this type of skin. Clay can be tolerated only if it is adjusted with soothing ingredients such as hydrosols or oil, and should be washed off before it dries. Blue clay is ideal, but hard to find.

TONER: Hydrosols are the most gentle, but aloe vera also may be used.

MOISTURIZER: Couperose skin may be present in any skin type, so choose your moisturizer accordingly and add appropriate essential oils.

ESSENTIAL OILS: Use gentle chamomile (Roman or German) to reduce inflammation, soothe delicate skin tissue, strengthen weak capillaries and reduce facial puffiness. The essential oils of helichrysum, Tanacetum annuum, rose, orange, neroli and lavender are very gentle and quite effective.

HERBS: Good herbal treatments to soothe broken capillaries include calendula, St. John's wort and comfrey as tea, or oil infusions used externally. Astringent herbal rinses made from oak bark and witch hazel can help unless your skin is very dry. Hawthorne and ginkgo taken internally can improve capillary strength from the inside. Other beneficial herbs are those high in flavonoids, such as St. John's wort and calendula. Foods high in flavonoids include buckwheat and peppers. Green tea contains an important type of tannin called *catechin*. According to a Russian report tea catechins strengthen capillaries. Tannin-rich green tea also makes a good last rinse in a facial treatment.

Mature Skin

As one matures, the complexion tends to become drier. Lines of character and wisdom become more apparent, although they are not always appreciated. The production of hormones that keep skin supple and radiant decreases with age. Skin produces less oil and fewer natural moisturizing factors, so skin treatments need to be adjusted with maturity. Those with fair complexions or a too-thin layer of fat under the skin, as well as those who smoke cigarettes, have a greater chance of developing wrinkles early.

At what age do we achieve mature skin? Some skin specialists say anyone over 25 has mature skin, but it is usually defined when lines start to form around the eyes or mouth. Many women begin noticing fine lines on the face at about 30 years of age, but it is never too early to start taking preventive measures. Antioxidant vitamins and limited sun exposure are the most effective defenses against aging of the skin.

The French beauty Ninon de L'Enclcs bitterly complained, "If God had to give woman wrinkles, He might at least have put them on the soles of her feet." Unfortunately, our youth-oriented society has not permitted women to feel comfortable about the aging process. If we can learn to love and accept ourselves and appreciate the wisdom that comes with experience and maturity, this situation will undoubtedly change. To treat mature skin, follow the recommendations for dry skin.

ESSENTIAL OILS: The essential oils of lavender, geranium, neroli, rosemary and rose are historic "anti-aging" ingredients for mature skin. Jasmine, frankincense, myrrh, carrot seed, helichrysum and cistus also rejuvenate this skin type by encouraging the formation of new cells. Rose hip seed oil offers additional benefits.

HERBS: Useful herbs include gota kola, and emollient herbs such as marshmallow and comfrey.

Sun-Damaged Skin

Sun damage can occur at any age, but the effects on the skin, especially premature wrinkling and pigmentation problems, become most apparent as we grow older. If you want to see sun damage on your skin before it is noticeable, look at your face through the light of a "Woods lamp." Some cosmetic counters have this device available as a service to their customers—and to sell products. If you've spent a lot of time in the sun, you will probably be shocked at what the lamp reveals. Most apparent are pigmentation irregularities that may show up later in life.

Cells called melanocytes, found in the basal layer of skin, contain a dark pigment. These cells differ from others because of the long, hollow arms that radiate from them. When stimulated by sunlight, these arms attach to neighboring skin cells and inject melanin into them. The result is that the coloration of the skin deepens into what we call a tan to protect sensitive underlying cells from the destructive effects of the sun. But melanin offers only so much protection, and after a few days of repeated sun exposure, the skin thickens in defense.

As always, prevention is the key. The most important measure to take is to limit your exposure to the sun, which is thought to be accountable for as much as 90 percent of skin aging. In fact, about 70 percent of sun damage occurs without our even trying: it happens as we walk down the street, ride a bike or drive a car. The long ultraviolet rays (called UVA) that penetrate into the skin's lower layers are particularly destructive and harm collagen, elastin and the DNA of the cell. These "aging rays" are present during all daylight hours, and they tend to increase susceptibility to the shorter UVB rays that tan surface skin. (These are strongest at midday.) Both types are associated with premature aging and skin cancer. UVC rays (very short ultraviolet rays) are thought to be the ones most responsible for the worldwide increase in skin cancer. With the depletion of the earth's protective ozone layer, every skin type needs protection from the sun's harmful rays.

Margaret Kripke, M.D., of the Anderson Cancer Center in Houston, Texas, says that sunscreen users may be spending long hours in the sun with a "false sense of security." Kripke thinks that immune suppression caused by ultraviolet light is not stopped by sunscreen. But rather than "Stop wearing sunscreen," her message is "Wear sunscreen and protective clothing, and minimize time in the sun." Although no natural ingredients have yet been found to fully protect us from the sun's rays, minimal sun protection can be obtained from a few natural products. Commercial sunscreens also use derivatives from natural products such as PABA, part of the B vitamin complex, and cinoxate, or cinnamic acid, from cinnamon. But questions about the safety of these and other chemical sunscreens raise concern; many reportedly cause allergic reactions. A new sunscreen from amino acids found in sea algae is currently being tested in Australia.

Research shows that sesame oil decreases the impact of the sun's burning rays by about 30 percent. Olive, coconut and peanut oils, along with aloe vera, block out a good 20 percent. Helichrysum essential oil also screens ultraviolet rays. (Use a 2-percent dilution.) The Xienta Institute for Skin Research in Bernville, Pennsylvania reports that vitamin E in a 5-percent dilution not only reduces burning, but retards cell damage to underlying skin by decreasing oxidation. At this point, we still advise using chemical sunscreens—at least on your face if you spend much time outdoors. Sunscreens sold at natural-food stores probably contain the least amount of artificial ingredients.

Phytotherapist Paul Duraffourd points out the cleansing virtues of carrot-seed oil, as well as its "positive effect on abscesses, ulcers, and even on epithelial cancers." Carrot-seed oil can be used to treat cellular irregularities such as moles. A study done in 1990 shows that caraway is anticarcinogenic when used topically. There is evidence that the same is true for citrus oils (which also have photosensitizing effects, so we are not recommending these oils for this purpose until more is learned about them.)

For a facial routine, follow the directions for dry skin. Sun-damaged skin also benefits from many of the suggestions for mature skin.

ESSENTIAL OILS: Lavender oil in a 2-percent dilution of aloe-vera gel is the best sunburn remedy. When stored in the refrigerator, this remedy provides cool, soothing relief for any burn. Rough skin patches, skin damaged by sun or prone to early wrinkles, and even precancerous areas respond especially well to a 3-percent dilution of carrot seed and caraway essential oils applied at least two times a day.

HERBS: Oils infused with St. John's wort, calendula, elder or comfrey ease sunburn. Even though some herb books say that St. John's wort causes skin photosensitivity when taken internally, there are no scientifically documented reports of this happening, except in cattle! When applying herbal oils to burns, wait until the "heat" has gone from the burn; vegetable oils applied to fresh burns can make them feel hotter. Use the aloe-lavender solution first, then apply the oils after a few days.

CREATING YOUR OWN SKIN-CARE PRODUCTS

Facial products are easy and fun to make in your own kitchen, and they can be prepared with minimal cost and fuss. They make great gifts at holidays, birthdays or just anytime. After many years of experimenting and teaching herbal cosmetic classes, we are glad to share some of our favorite recipes with you. Remember to label and date your creations so that your calendula face cream is not mistaken for mayonnaise by some unfortunate family member. (We speak from experience.)

Here are a few recipes for each step of a facial routine. Use these ideas and the ingredients for your skin type to make up your own. If you do not have time to make your own cosmetics, increase the effectiveness of commercial products by adding essential oils. Just be sure to look for good-quality products that contain no mineral oil, synthetic colors and scents, or other potentially harmful ingredients. (Refer to skin care sections for specific herb and essential ingredient suggestions.)

Cleansers

Dry-Skin Cleansing Solution

1/4 cup hydrosol or aloe gel
1 teaspoon vegetable oil
1 teaspoon glycerin
1/2 teaspoon grapefruit-seed extract
5 drops rosemary verbenone essential oil

Shake well before each use—this solution foams in the bottle, but does not lather on the skin. Aloe gel makes a thicker solution than the hydrosol. Apply with fingers or cotton pads, then rinse.

Oily-Skin Cleansing Solution

1/4 cup hydrosol or witch hazel
1 teaspoon herbal vinegar
1 teaspoon glycerin
1/2 teaspoon grapefruit-seed extract
1 teaspoon echinacea tincture (for acne)
5 drops eucalyptus

Follow instructions above for dry-skin cleanser.

Exfoliants

Facial Scrub

1 part oatmeal
1/3 part cornmeal
sprinkle of clay (optional)
1/3 part herbs (lavender and peppermint)

Grind ingredients in an electric coffee grinder. Store powder in a closed container. To use the scrub, make a paste of 1 teaspoon scrub powder and enough water or hydrosol to moisten, and apply to a dampened face. Gently scrub face and rinse with warm water. This mixture can also be used as a mask—just leave it on for 10 minutes.

Herbal Scrub for Teenage Skin

1/4 cup oatmeal
1 tablespoon dry lavender
1 tablespoon dry thyme leaves
1 tablespoon dry rosemary leaves
5 drops tea tree essential oil

Grind oatmeal and herbs into a fine powder in an electric coffee grinder. Add essential oil and mix well. Store dry in an airtight jar. To use, moisten 1 teaspoon of the scrub with rosewater or aloe. Gently scrub and rinse.

Facial Steams

The Basic Recipe

1 quart boiling water
a large handful of herbs (refer to your skin type)
5 drops essential oils (refer to your skin type)

Steep herbs for 5 to 10 minutes, covered. Remove the lid and add essential oils; leave the herbs in the water at this stage. Make a tent with a towel over the pot and steam for up to 10 minutes. Strain the herbs and save the tea for the final rinse water at the end of the facial.

Facial Masks

Mask for Dry Skin

1 tablespoon facial scrub
1 teaspoon vegetable oil
1 teaspoon honey
1 tablespoon rosewater or aloe juice
1 drop rose essential oil
1 egg yolk (optional)

Neroli essential oil is also wonderful here. Mix the ingredients and apply to the face. Leave mask on for 5 to 10 minutes. Rinse.

Mask for Oily Skin

1 tablespoon clay
1 tablespoon witch hazel
1 strawberry, mashed
1 drop spike lavender essential oil

Mix ingredients together and apply, leaving mask on for 5 to 10 minutes. Rinse.

Mask for Acne Skin

1 tablespoon bentonite clay (or other facial clay)
2 tablespoons comfrey-leaf tea
1 teaspoon ground elder flowers
1 teaspoon ground strawberry leaves
1 drop lavender essential oil

Make comfrey-leaf tea by steeping 1 tablespoon dried comfrey leaves in 1/2 cup water. Let cool and mix ingredients into a paste. Apply to face in a thin layer, avoiding the area around the eyes. Leave on for 10 to 15 minutes, or as long as is comfortable. Rinse. Use the leftover tea as a final compress or rinse.

Intensive Treatment for Acne

1/2 teaspoon powdered goldenseal root
1/4 teaspoon tea-tree essential oil

Combine ingredients into a paste, adding water if necessary to obtain the right consistency, and apply directly to acne spots. Let dry and remain on the skin for at least 20 minutes. Rinse.

Mask for Combination Skin

1 tablespoon yogurt
1 tablespoon applesauce
1 tablespoon papaya, mashed
2 drops liquid lecithin (optional)
1 drop geranium essential oil

Blend ingredients together. Apply to face for at least 5 minutes. Rinse.

Exfoliating Mask for All Skin Types

2 tablespoons mashed papaya
1 teaspoon honey
1 drop carrot-seed oil
1 tablespoon powdered peppermint leaf (or enough to firm mixture)

Mix, apply and leave on skin for at least 10 minutes. Rinse.

Toners

Toner for Oily or Problem Skin

1/2 cup witch hazel
1/2 cup chopped fresh herbs, or 1/4 cup crumbled dry herbs
2 tablespoons rose water or aloe vera
5 drops each cedarwood and lavender essential oils

Soak the herbs and witch hazel together for 10 days. Strain and add the rosewater or aloe and the essential oils. Shake well before each use.

Toner for Dry or Mature Skin

2 ounces aloe-vera gel
2 ounces orange-blossom water
1 teaspoon infused calendula vinegar
5 drops helichrysum essential oil
800 IUs vitamin E oil

Combine the ingredients and shake before use.

Toner for Delicate or Couperose Skin

1/4 cup aloe-vera juice
1/4 cup rose water
1/4 teaspoon glycerin
5 drops each neroli and rose essential oils

Combine ingredients and shake well before using. Apply with cotton swabs or mist the skin with a sprayer.

Fragrant Waters

10 drops essential oil
4 ounces distilled water

Shake well before each use. Store in a glass spray bottle. May be used on the entire body.

Creams and Lotions

Although it may seem complicated, it is really quite simple to make creams and lotions in your own kitchen. The process requires a bit of patience and preparation, but with a little experience you'll be inspired by the results.

Get familiar with the ingredients that are used in lotions and creams, with how they can change your product and benefit your skin. This introduction to the subject addresses some of the questions most commonly put to us by students throughout our years of teaching natural cosmetics. You may want to start out simply, using plain oil, water and beeswax. After you've mastered the processing technique, you can experiment with the "extras"—different colors, waters and oils to give you more variation in your lotion recipes. Refer to other chapters to acquaint yourself with unfamiliar ingredients.

Preservatives

There is no need for preservatives in homemade products using dry ingredients, such as facial scrubs, bath salts or powders; however, creams, lotions or anything containing water carry a personal invitation for bacterial growth. Even dipping clean fingers into homemade cosmetics contributes to such growth, so it's best to use a small cosmetic spatula or clean chopstick to scoop creams from the jar. With squeeze bottles, you don't need to scoop out the product; they work well for a thin lotion, but creams are too thick to pass through the narrow necks.

The best preservatives for your products are the essential oils. Some of the most effective ones are lavender, benzoin and eucalyptus, but essential oils are antibacterial or antifungal to some degree. Consider their individual properties and odors when choosing the most suitable oils for your creations. Under most conditions, adding essential oils assures a six-month shelf life for lotions and creams. With refrigeration, most products keep at least three times as long. To keep products longer, you can also add 400 IUs of vitamin E to the oil portion, or dissolve 1/4 teaspoon of vitamin C crystals in the water portion. Grapefruit seed extract, although not an essential oil, is a powerful antibacterial agent; add 5-10 drops to a recipe, at the same time as you add the essential oils. We have never encountered spoilage with a lotion containing at least 2-percent essential oil, even after it was stored for a year or more at room temperature. Start production with clean tools, including the blender, bowls and measuring cups, and be fastidious about wiping jar lids after every use of your product.

Emulsifiers

Emulsifiers bind water and oil together so they will not separate. Chemical emulsifiers slightly reduce the penetrating power of essential oils, which are more likely to remain in the product than to search out the oil medium of the skin. Since all lotions and creams need some emulsification, we have chosen the most natural ones: beeswax, lanolin, glycerin and lecithin. We've included general guidelines to follow when you're feeling creative and want to design your own products. We came up with these proportions through trial and error, and we want to save you the error part!

Beeswax

Beeswax is the most common natural emulsifier for homemade cosmetics, the best for holding water and oil in suspension. It can slightly thicken a lotion or harden a lip balm, depending on how much is added. After beekeepers have extracted the honey, they melt the comb, strain it and pour it into blocks. Beeswax is sold at craft, natural-food and herb stores, and by beekeepers. Be sure you are not buying paraffin or impure beeswax. If beeswax is brittle, it is probably old. If it is dark, it may contain propolis, an antibacterial material used by bees to seal their hives. A bit of propolis in your beeswax is fine for cosmetics (although it may leave dark specks), and because it is very antibacterial it may even extend the shelf life. Propolis is also sold separately, but will not work as a substitute for beeswax.

For 1 cup base oil, use up to 3/4 ounce (by weight) beeswax to make a salve, 3/4 ounce for lip balm, up to 3/4 ounce to make cream, and up to 1/2 ounce to thicken lotion. The minimum amount of beeswax that I have successfully used in a lotion recipe is 12 grams.

Lanolin

This is the oil that is removed from sheep's wool. In structure, it is much like the oil of our own skin glands and thus is easily absorbed. There are three types of lanolin. Thick anhydrous lanolin (without water) is the least desirable, because it does not mix well with water. Hydrous lanolin contains a little water, is much easier to work with, and can be used in making lotions. The third type, liquid lanolin, is designed for use as a lotion on its own, but it can also be used as an ingredient for lotions and creams.

Oil-rich lanolin makes a product more emollient and slightly thicker, but too much of it can make the product sticky. However, this may be just what is needed in a water-resistant diaper-rash cream or salve intended to adhere well to the skin. A small amount of lanolin will help emulsify a cream or lotion, but don't rely on it alone to thicken the product. The formula will still require beeswax.

Lanolin is sold at most drugstores, but be sure to smell it before purchasing; some smells so strongly of sheep that no amount of essential oil can cover the odor. Stir it into slightly warmed ingredients in the oil portion of your creams. Liquid lanolin can be added to the water portion in the blender.

Use up to 1/2 teaspoon of hydrous or liquid lanolin to enrich 1 cup of base oil. Some people have a sensitivity to lanolin, so test a small amount on the skin before using it in products, especially in those made for babies.

Glycerin

Glycerin is a clear, sweet, sticky product derived from plants or animals, or made synthetically. It is often a by-product of soap-making. The more expensive "vegetable" glycerin comes from coconut or olive-oil soap, instead of from the more common tallow and lard soaps.

Glycerin is a humectant, meaning that it absorbs water from its surroundings. A little goes a long way, and if you use too much it makes a product very sticky. Because glycerin will draw moisture from the air, it works wonderfully as a moisturizing ingredient, especially if you live in a humid climate.

Glycerin is also a natural preservative and will mix with either water or oil. This makes it a good emulsifier, but don't rely on it alone to thicken your creams or to hold ingredients in suspension. Glycerin has a long history of use in cosmetic products. Among the most popular glycerin products are "Rose Water and Glycerin" lotion and "Pa's Cornhusker's Lotion," both manufactured since the early part of this century.

Use up to 1 teaspoon of glycerin per cup of cosmetic base.

Lecithin

This emulsifier is derived from soybeans, and also is found in egg yolk, once commonly used to emulsify bath and hair products. It increases the spreadability of a product and leaves the skin feeling very smooth, although using too much can make it sticky. Sold at health-food stores, lecithin comes in granules or liquid form. It can be used in creams or lotions.

Use up to 1/2 teaspoon granulated or liquid lecithin to 1 cup oil base. It is not water-soluble, and is best added when melting oils and beeswax.

Colors

It's fun to color lotions, creams, bath salts and other products. Experiment with the various possibilities, mixing and matching to develop attractive shades. Green, red and yellow are easily derived from natural plant pigments; blue and violet shades are trickier. The best way to add color is to use a carrier oil that has been infused with a colorful herb. For example, calendula and turmeric produce a rich yellow; comfrey, plantain, nettle and chickweed oil provide a nice green; and alkanet is a gorgeous pink to red, depending on how strong you make it. Blue shades are much more difficult to achieve naturally. We have experimented with essential oils such as *Tanacetum annuum* and German chamomile, both of which contain vivid blue chamazulene. Although the smell was incredible, the amount needed to make the lotion blue made it very costly. There was one more drawback: the color was bright to begin with, but soon changed to a gray-blue color that evolved into a muddy green in a few weeks. Still, if money is no object and you plan on using the lotion quickly, you'll love it!

The color of the vegetable oil itself will also influence the color of your final product. Unrefined safflower oil is yellow; extra virgin olive oil is green. Herb tea or an infused vinegar, witch hazel or tincture used as part of the water base in creams and lotions can lend some color, but the change is less dramatic. A colorless oil and plain water result in a very nice white cream or lotion.

Extras

The addition of special ingredients—such as bee pollen, royal jelly, herbal extracts, honey or glycerin—will set your lotions apart. These ingredients contain vitamins, minerals and enzymes beneficial to the skin. Herbal extracts can be added in tincture or tea form in the water part of your recipe. Small amounts of these boosters, one teaspoon or less, will be sufficient to benefit your creams and lotions.

Water and Oil

The basis of creams and lotions is water and oil. These ingredients can be mixed and matched to meet the needs of any skin type. The water portion of your recipe can be any one, or a combination, of the ingredients in the water list below; the same holds true for the oil list. Just be sure to maintain the proper proportion of water to oil in a recipe. All lotions and creams will become firmer as they cool, so it is easier to pour them into wide-mouth jars as soon as they are done. If you use a saturated oil, such as cocoa butter or coconut, the product will be even firmer when cold, but will melt readily when applied to the skin.

Water	Oil
distilled water	any vegetable oil
spring water	herbal oil infusion
aloe-vera juice	cocoa butter
rose water or other hydrosols	coconut oil

Tools Needed to Make Creams and Lotions

You probably already have all of these items in your own kitchen. Make sure everything is squeaky-clean before you begin.

blender	small saucepan
rubber spatula	jars
chopstick	wide-mouth funnel (optional)
Pyrex measuring cup (1 cup)	

Recipes

Note: Follow the "Basic Cream" directions for the cream or lotion recipe given below. Do not try to cut these recipes in half. There will not be enough liquid for the blender blades to work with, and the mixture will not always thicken sufficiently.

Basic Cream

1 cup oil
3/4 ounce beeswax (22 grams)
1 cup water (lukewarm)
30-50 drops essential oils

Add shaved beeswax to the oil in a Pyrex measuring cup. Set the Pyrex cup in a small saucepan of simmering water that reaches halfway up the side of the measuring cup. Heat just until the beeswax melts, and remove the measuring cup from the pan. Cool for a few minutes, but not long enough for the beeswax to harden. You should be able to put your finger in the oil without discomfort, and a film of hardened beeswax should form at the edge. Put the lid on your blender and remove the center ring. The use of a wide-mouth funnel will help reduce splattering. Pour the water into the blender through the funnel, turn the blender on high speed and slowly add the oil-beeswax mixture. This is just like making mayonnaise; proper emulsion and consistency will depend not only on the temperature of the oil mixture, but also on how steadily the oil is poured into the water. This is not an exact science, however, and there is a fair amount of compensation for both criteria, so don't panic.

The whole concoction should begin to harden after about three-quarters of the oil has been added. The chopstick is a handy tool at this point if you need to stir the ingredients as you pour. Be careful to stir only on the top edges, not deep in the center where the blades are. Add the rest of the oil slowly, until the mixture becomes too stiff to take any more oil or until all the water is incorporated—which doesn't always happen. Sometimes there is a little water left in the blender; pour it off, or carefully absorb it from the edges with a tissue.

You should now have a thick, beautiful cream. Add the essential oils last, turning on the blender just enough to incorporate the oils, being careful not to overblend the mixture. It will usually take 30 to 50 drops (1/4 to 1/2 teaspoon) of essential oil to scent this quantity of cream, but personal preference will dictate the amount. Using the rubber spatula, scoop or pour the cream, depending on its thickness, into wide-mouth (1- to 2-ounce) jars. Extra cream is best stored in the refrigerator to prolong shelf life.

Basic Lotion

3/4 cup oil
1 cup water
1/2 ounce beeswax, shaved (about 2 tablespoons)
30 drops essential oils

Follow the directions above.

Exotic Rose Cream

1 cup rose water
1 tablespoon tincture of rose petals
2 ounces rosehip-seed oil
2 ounces macadamia-nut oil
1 ounce squalene or jojoba oil
1 ounce alkanet oil
15 grams beeswax (1/2 ounce)
800 IUs vitamin E
20 drops rose oil

Follow the directions above. A luxury for all skin types!

Natural Sun Oil

2 ounces sesame oil
2 ounces calendula oil
2 ounces aloe-vera gel
1 teaspoon vitamin E oil
8 drops each lavender and carrot essential oils

Combine ingredients. Shake well before using. Remember, this will not provide much sun protection. It makes a good oil after sun exposure.

10

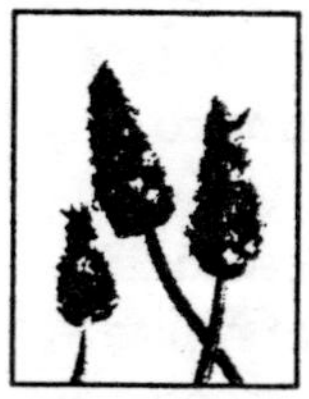

Essential Oils in the Kitchen

There is no reason to confine yourself to the cosmetic and therapeutic applications of essential oils and aromatic hydrosols. Aromatics are wonderful in the kitchen, and with a bit of experience, a few guidelines and a creative mind, the culinary possibilities are endless.

Culinary herbs have always been a mainstay of creative cooking, adding flavor, color and nutritional value to recipes. But have you ever considered topping a geranium sponge pudding with a dollop of neroli whipped cream, dreamed of scented sorbets, or imagined real rose ice cream? Iced herbal tea with a splash of aromatic hydrosol is heavenly on a hot summer day! Or how about flavoring your favorite jar of black tea or your sugar bowl with a few drops of essential oil? Try oil of dill in potato salad, or caraway oil in cream cheese. Reading this chapter and trying a few of the recipes should elevate your cooking creations to new heights of inspiration.

Safety is an important consideration in the kitchen, as it is with any aspect of aromatherapy. Be sure you use pure oils from reliable sources, not synthetic scents or flavorings. Essential oils extracted with carbon dioxide are ideal for culinary use because their flavor is often truer to the plant. Absolutes are never used in the kitchen, because of the solvent residues that may be left as a by-product of the extraction process. In general, it is wise to use only those oils that you would normally think of as foods—for example, citruses or seed oils such as anise, dill, celery, cumin and coriander. Also suitable are essential oils from flowers and medicinal herbs such as rose, neroli, geranium, lemon verbena, mint and melissa. (All of these taste great in bubbly water.) Then there are the essential oils from common spices—ginger, cinnamon, clove, nutmeg, cardamom and black pepper, to name just a few. Oils from commonly used culinary herbs—thyme, rosemary, oregano, savory, marjoram and sage—are great for savory dishes, but their bitter or overpowering flavors are a bit tricky to work with.

Essential oils, which evaporate as food is heated, yield their best flavor and aroma uncooked. It is best to use the oils in fresh-food dishes such as salad dressings, cold soups, blender drinks and uncooked desserts. In cooked dishes like soups and sauces, add the oils at the last minute; only a few drops are necessary. With casseroles, cakes and other baked dishes, you may need to add a bit more essential oil to compensate for evaporation. Nothing is more important than dosage—except quality, which we're assuming is good. Experiment, but be conservative until you get the feel of how essential oils flavor food. Start with one drop, and go from there. (A little bit really does go a long way; consider that it takes 30 to 60 roses to make one precious drop of rose oil.)

EXTRACTS

Making your own flavoring extracts from essential oils is easy, economical and a good way to reduce dosage when one drop of an essential oil is too much. Any culinary essential oil can be made into an extract, but the technique is especially appropriate for oils that are harsh, strongly flavored or very expensive.

The usual carrier for commercial extracts is alcohol, but vegetable glycerin and vegetable oil are perfectly suitable, and mix better with essential oils. Glycerin is sweet and soluble in most mediums. I [Mindy] have been making my own rose extract for years, and have found that glycerin is the best carrier for this particular essential oil. Alcohol works well with the citrus oils and peppermint. Use olive oil for savory extracts. Shake all extracts before using. Start with 5 drops of essential oil per ounce of carrier. Adjust to suit your taste. Use 1/2 to 1 teaspoon per recipe.

AROMATIC HONEYS

This is a delightful way to introduce even the staunchest skeptic to the pleasures of essential oils. Essential oils from herbs, spices, seeds and flowers make excellent honeys. Favorites include angelica, ginger, cardamom, rose, peppermint and bergamot. You can use the oils individually or in combination: peppermint and ginger, rosemary and lemon, cinnamon and orange are compatible flavors. Aromatic honeys are perfect for flavoring coffee or tea, and are effective digestive aids taken after a meal. They are also very handy for making instant tea when traveling; just add one teaspoon honey to a cup of hot water and enjoy. I prefer to use a light honey, but dark honeys work fine.

Honeys will keep forever, but some may crystallize. To reliquify, loosen the lid and place the jar in hot water until the honey melts. Never heat honeys in the microwave.

Aromatic Honey

1/4 cup honey
1-2 drops essential oil

Begin with one drop; it is usually enough. Stir well.

AROMATIC HYDROSOLS

Aromatic hydrosols also add flair in the kitchen. Many gourmet or traditional ethnic cookbooks call for rose water or orange-blossom water in exotic dishes, but imagine using lemon-verbena water or rosemary water in some of your own recipes. Hydrosols are much milder in flavor than essential oils and are safer (as long as the plant they are derived from is nontoxic). There is little information on the medicinal uses of hydrosols, but it is known that the Romans drank rose water for a hangover. Hydrosols are best kept refrigerated.

The following recipes should help get you started and spark your own ideas for creating exotic culinary delights. With a little inspiration, you can dramatically dress up and add excitement to almost any recipe.

Hydrosols are easily added to many recipes, and you are limited only by what is available. It is safe to ingest an ounce or two of an aromatic hydrosol at one sitting, but you will find that you do not need nearly that much for flavoring. Rose and orange blossom, frequently called for in Middle Eastern recipes, are the most readily available hydrosols and can often be found in your supermarket or gourmet deli. Be sure you are not using an artificially scented water, or a product loaded with preservatives or emulsifiers. Hydrosols, like essential oils, are best used in recipes that require no cooking. Always taste a hydrosol before adding it to a recipe; some hydrosols taste burned or overcooked. (A hydrosol suitable for flavoring should be fragrant and fresh.) One tablespoon of hydrosol is plenty to flavor a cup of water, but you will notice the fragrance and flavor with just a sprinkle. Try hydrosols in bubbly water or champagne.

Lavender Lemonade

2 cups prepared lemonade
1-2 tablespoons lavender hydrosol

Combine ingredients. For a special touch add ice made with fresh lavender flowers frozen into the cubes.

Refreshing Mint Julep

2 cups water
1/2 cup fresh peppermint leaves
2 tablespoons lemon-verbena hydrosol

Rub the peppermint leaves to release the essential oils; soak them in cold water overnight and strain. Add hydrosol and serve with ice cubes with whole fresh borage flowers frozen inside.

Orange Rosemary Sorbet

1/4 cup water
2 tablespoons honey
2 cups fresh-squeezed orange juice
1/2 teaspoon finely chopped fresh rosemary leaves
2 tablespoons rosemary hydrosol

Gently warm water and honey together until the honey melts. Add orange juice, hydrosol and rosemary leaves. Churn in ice-cream maker and serve in chilled bowls for a refreshing fat-free dessert.

Peach Blush

3 ripe peaches
1 cup plain yogurt
2 tablespoons honey
4 ice cubes
1-2 drops mandarin essential oil

Mix everything together in a blender. Start with one drop of essential oil and taste before adding a second.

Jitterbug-Perfume Spritzer

1/2 cup strawberries
2 tablespoons honey
1/2 tablespoon beet juice
1 teaspoon bee pollen
4 fresh melissa (or peppermint) leaves
2 cups mineral water
1 drop melissa essential oil

Blend all ingredients and serve with a fresh jasmine blossom in each glass. If you don't have the beet juice, soak 1/4 cup grated beets in the mineral water for 10 minutes and strain. (This recipe was inspired by Tom Robbins' novel *Jitterbug Perfume*.)

Strawberry-Rose Ice Cream

1 cup fresh strawberries
3 tablespoons nonfat dry milk powder
1/4-1/3 cup honey
3/4 cup plain yogurt
1 cup heavy cream
1-2 drops rose essential oil

Mix all ingredients in the blender until smooth. Churn in an ice-cream maker until frozen. When my children tasted this they thought it was "too perfumey." (I absolutely love rose, so I thought it was "to die for.") You may want to try just one drop of rose oil the first time you make this.

AROMATIC WHIPPED CREAM

If you really want to impress and delight your dinner guests, you'll try this idea from herbalist and aromatherapy enthusiast Diana DeLuca, who serves a neroli whipped cream that is out of this world. I [Mindy] was so taken with the topping I can't remember what it was served on; since then, I've discovered that it is great with chocolate desserts. I have also experimented with other essential oils and had many pleasant results. Cardamom whipped cream on gingerbread is fabulous, or as an exotic topping for cappuccino or hot chocolate. How about black-currant whipped cream atop apple cobbler? Mandarin cream on angel-food cake?

For a low-fat topping, add essential oils to yogurt.

Whipping Cream

1/2 pint whipping cream
1-2 drops essential oil

Whip cream to desired consistency, add essential oil and mix well. Start with one drop only. Add sweetener if desired.

Quick, easy and pleasing to children of all ages. The digestive attributes of peppermint are so good, you could call this a medicinal dessert.

Peppermint Tapioca

3 tablespoons quick-cooking tapioca
2 3/4 cups milk
1/3 cup honey
1 egg (optional)
1 square (1 ounce) semisweet chocolate (optional)
1-2 drops peppermint oil

Mix together everything except the peppermint oil, and let the tapioca soak for 10 minutes. Cook over medium heat, stirring until the chocolate is melted. Bring to a boil, lower heat and add the beaten egg slowly so it won't curdle. Cook 5 minutes longer. Let cool 15 minutes. Add peppermint oil to taste and pour into dessert cups. Serve warm or cold.

Present the following suggestive delights to your lover on a warm, sultry night!

Midnight at the Oasis Balls

1 cup hulled sesame seeds
2 tablespoons tahini or almond butter
2-3 tablespoons honey
1 tablespoon finely chopped dates
1 teaspoon cardamom powder
1 teaspoon bee pollen
1/2 teaspoon ginseng powder (optional)
1/2 teaspoon vanilla extract
1 drop rose oil

Grind the seeds in an electric coffee grinder. Add the rose oil to the vanilla to help with dispersal. Mix all ingredients thoroughly and form into balls. Roll in shredded coconut, cocoa powder or whole sesame seeds. Refrigerate and serve at just the right moment!

The addition of geranium oil in this low-fat dessert adds a delightful floral hint.

Lemon Geranium Sponge Cake

1/3 cup honey
3 tablespoons flour
1/4 cup fresh lemon juice
1 teaspoon grated lemon peel
2 eggs, separated
1 cup milk
5 drops geranium oil

Preheat oven to 325°F. Beat together honey, lemon juice, rind and flour. After adding yolks, milk and geranium oil, mix again. In a separate bowl, beat egg whites until stiff, then fold into the lemon mixture. Pour into a buttered 8-inch-square baking pan or in individual custard cups. If available, place fresh rose geranium leaves on top of the pudding. Bake in a hot water bath for 45 to 50 minutes until the cake is set and the knife comes out clean. Serve warm or cold.

French Toast with Flair

2 eggs
1/2 cup of milk
1 tablespoon pure maple syrup
1 drop cinnamon-bark essential oil

Mix all the wet ingredients well and soak the bread thoroughly before frying. Bergamot, anise or cardamom are nice substitutes for the cinnamon oil. Cinnamon is strong, so if you find one drop too much for your palate, try one teaspoon of homemade essential-oil extracts or dilute with more milk.

OTHER SAVORY RECIPES

Using flavored vegetable oils is a great way to tone down the strong flavor of essential oils such as thyme, oregano, basil, savory, rosemary and sage. Sometimes just one drop of these oils is too much, especially for light flavoring or when making small portions, so having a prepared dilution is handy. Flavored oils are nice for making croutons, as a base for salad dressings, and for basting grilled vegetables and fish. Essential oil of lemon in olive oil makes a delicious marinade or dip for french bread.

Vegetable oils make a better carrier for savory extracts than glycerin or alcohol because they tone down the harshness of these oils better than any other carrier. Olive oil serves very nicely as a carrier for food flavoring, but you can use canola, sesame, safflower, flax or other vegetable oils instead. Combine four drops of an essential oil (or combination of oils) to one ounce of vegetable oil. Use 1/2 teaspoon or more (to taste) of the prepared oil in any recipe. For a lighter flavoring, use less essential oil or make an infused oil from the herb itself. Whenever possible, add these flavorings just before serving. It is best to store them in the refrigerator.

The following dressing is especially good on organic baby greens, with lightly toasted hazelnuts and gorgonzola cheese.

Herbed Vinaigrette Dressing

1/4 cup balsamic vinegar
1/2 cup olive oil
2 tablespoons water
1 teaspoon honey
1 teaspoon prepared Dijon mustard
1 clove garlic
1/4 teaspoon salt
2 drops black-pepper oil
4 drops basil oil
2 drops thyme oil

Mix everything together in the blender. Pour onto salad and toss well.

The addition of wild garden greens and herbs makes the following soup a real immunity booster.

Wild Miso Soup

1 cup leafy wild greens (dandelion, dock, mustard, lamb's quarters, mustard, mallow)
1 onion
1 carrot
3 shiitake mushrooms
(if dried, soak for 30 minutes in water)
1/4 cup lovage leaves
1 slice astragalus root
1 tablespoon ginseng rootlets
1 tablespoon fresh ginger
1 quart water
3 tablespoons dark miso
1 drop thyme essential oil diluted in 1 teaspoon vegetable oil (or 1 teaspoon flavored oil)

If you are not familiar with the wild weeds in your area, use chard or kale. The astragalus and ginseng rootlets can be purchased from an herb or natural-foods store.

Sauté chopped onion, carrot, mushrooms and ginger in a bit of olive oil for 5 minutes. Add chopped wild greens, lovage, astragalus, ginseng and water. Bring to a boil, cover, and simmer for about 20 minutes. Remove from heat. In a cup, thin the miso with a little soup stock, and add it to the pot. Add the diluted thyme oil, stir well and serve. If you reheat this soup, use low heat and watch it carefully; boiling destroys important enzymes in miso.

Essential Creamy Gazpacho

3 large fresh tomatoes, peeled and seeded
1/2 avocado
1 cup plain yogurt
1 cucumber, peeled and seeded
2 tablespoons fresh cilantro
2 tablespoons white wine
Juice of 1/2 lemon
1 clove garlic
1 green onion
1 tablespoon fresh mint leaves
1/2 teaspoon salt
Freshly ground pepper to taste
1-2 drops dill essential oil

Start by chopping the tomatoes in the blender. Add the other vegetables, wine, lemon juice and salt, and pulse just until everything is chunky. Add 1 drop of the essential oil, mix well and taste. Add another, if needed. Chill for at least one hour before serving. A cool treat on a hot summer day!

Savory Cheese Torta

Stunning creations suitable for centerpieces, tortas are as elegant as they are versatile.

1/3 cup sun-dried tomatoes
Whole basil leaves
8 ounces cream cheese, softened
2-3 drops sweet basil essential oil
1 teaspoon paprika
2 garlic cloves, pressed
3 tablespoons chopped chives
1/3 cup pine nuts, lightly toasted
8 ounces sharp cheddar, grated

Soak the dried tomatoes in hot water to soften, if needed; drain and chop. Line a two-cup bowl or other mold with two layers of cheesecloth. Arrange small basil leaves in a circular pattern in the bottom of the bowl. Stir the cream cheese into a smooth consistency, adding the basil essential oil, paprika, garlic and chives. Press half the cream-cheese mixture into the mold, being careful not to disturb the basil leaves. Add a layer of dried tomatoes, then the pine nuts. Layer in the grated cheddar and press lightly. Finish with the rest of the cream cheese. Fold the cheesecloth over the mixture, cover and refrigerate overnight. Before serving, unfold the cheesecloth from the top of the mold and invert the bowl onto a bed of lettuce. Lift off the bowl and carefully unwrap the cheesecloth.

This is a very versatile recipe. You can create a variety of tortas by using different cheeses and layering with chopped olives, pesto, marinated mushrooms or artichoke hearts, different nuts and herbs, and various essential oils. Go wild!

PART III

Alchemy

And so he would now study perfumes and the secrets of their manufacture.... He saw that there was no mood of the mind that had not its counterpart in the sensuous life, and set himself to discover their true relations... seeking often to elaborate the several influences of sweet-smelling roots, and scented pollen-laden flowers, or aromatic balms, and of dark and fragrant woods...

—Oscar Wilde, from The Picture of Dorian Gray

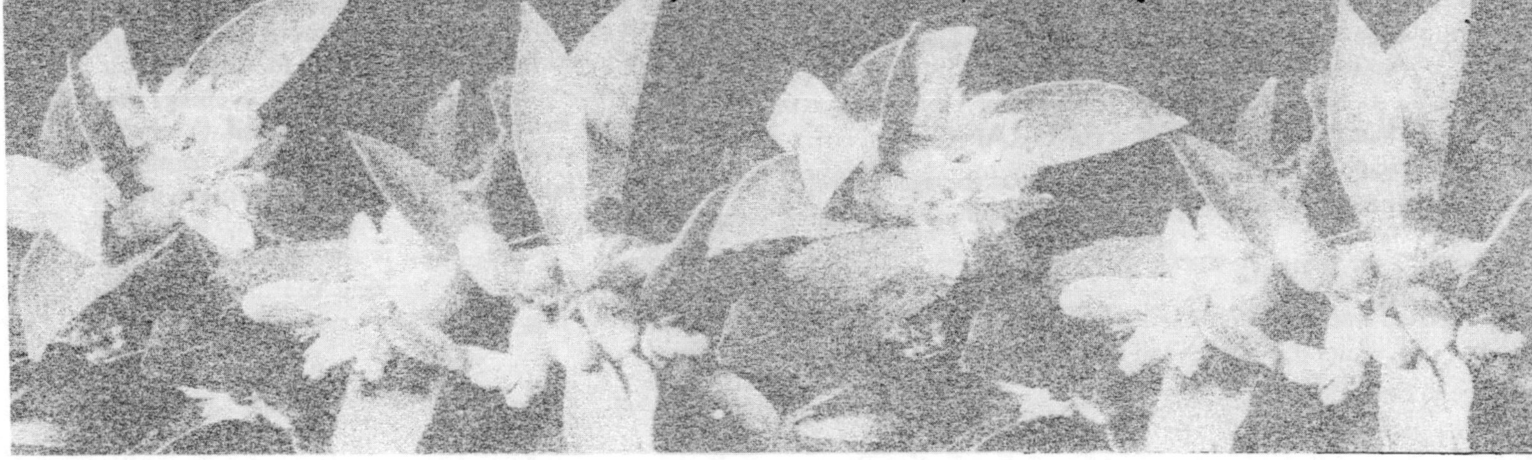

11

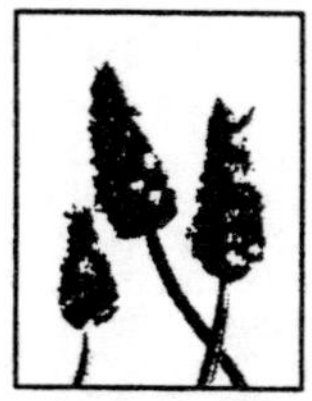

Blending Essential Oils—The Perfumer's Art

Blending—the art of combining a number of oils to create an appealing and interesting fragrance—can be a challenging, if not overwhelming, prospect for the beginning aromatherapist. However, anyone can learn to create wonderful combinations that are both effective and pleasant. All it takes is a basic understanding of a few elementary principles, and a bit of imagination.

Imagine that you are sniffing a single essential oil, such as lemon. The familiar smell is pleasant enough by itself, but it is very one-dimensional. Your brain responds, "Yes, this is lemon." But add the woodsy smell of cedarwood and the slightest hint of spearmint, and suddenly your nose is experiencing a whole bouquet of fragrances. Your one-dimensional fragrance has been expanded into a collage that will pique interest and continue to intrigue. This is the effect that perfumers strive for in creating their products: a blend of fragrances, too elusive to pin down, that keeps one coming back for more.

You will use the same blending techniques to create therapeutic formulas. Perfume-blending rules enhance the appeal of any aromatherapy product, whatever its intended use. As the Chinese say, "Every perfume is a medicine."

BLENDING FOR FRAGRANCE

Perfume has been used throughout the ages to influence mood or create an image. Inspiration can come from a variety of sources. The four seasons, certain times of day, favorite music or colors, or simple pleasant emotions can all lend themselves to the creation of a characteristic fragrance.

Representational perfumes have fragrances that remind one of a familiar substance such as a flower, leather or a fine tea blend. *Abstract perfumes* embody the feel, or rather the smell, of an experience. They suggest a time or an occasion: a hot summer day, calm before a thunderstorm, a picnic celebration, Christmas morning.

Resinous and aromatic gums and roots give us winterlike scents. Heavier perfumes are deep and sensuous. If you are more of a spring person, you may find yourself attracted to light, fresh scents such as geranium and lavender, whereas summer people go for fruity, rich scents such as the citruses and the sweet smell of ylang-ylang. Autumn types often are drawn to the herblike and pungent scents of clary sage or spicy black pepper.

The object of perfumery has always been to create a sense of intrigue and excitement around the wearer. Keep the mood light, fresh or fruity for the office, a party or a sports event. For a romantic evening, you may choose a heavy, warm, sensuous blend. (You will probably want to avoid wearing too much scent for any occasion, however; subtlety, after all, is much more mysterious.)

CLASSIFYING ODORS

Perfumers have developed a simple system of classification related to four kinds of odor sensations: fragrant (sweet), acid (sour), burnt (empyreumatic) and caprylic (oenanthic, which is generally perceived as unpleasant in itself, but interesting when used to add "color" to another class of scents). Other perfumers use the names commonly associated with the scent, such as minty, balsamic, fruity, rosaceous and spicy. Charles Piesse, in *The Art of Perfumery*, relates the odors to the octaves of a musical scale, theorizing that scents influence the olfactory nerves in much the same way that sounds influence the auditory nerves. As a musician harmonizes sound into a musical chord, so must a perfumer harmonize scent into a fragrant bouquet.

The array of synthetic fragrances available to the professional perfumer is somewhat overwhelming. Blending with pure plant oils simplifies the process of creating perfumes, if only because there are fewer materials to choose from. The following system categorizes natural fragrance ingredients in a practical way that will help you get started in creating harmonious essential-oil perfumes.

Perfume Categories

In this system, fragrances are divided into six main categories. Familiarity with these categories will enhance your ability to create your own unique blends, Please note that the denotations "F" and "M" refer to scents that have been traditionally designated "female" or "male," but don't let such preconceptions limit your choices.

Floral (F)—Individual or in combinations (bouquets). Examples include rose, jasmine, ylang-ylang and neroli (orange blossom). Popular perfumes in this group are White Shoulders, Arpege, Zen and L'Air du Temps.

Subgroups: fruity, fresh, sweet, green.

Oriental (F/M)—Heavy, with a dominant "animal," spicy or vanilla note. Examples include cinnamon, frankincense and patchouli. Many popular perfumes are oriental types, such as Tabu, Opium, Youth Dew and Shalimar.

Subgroups: sweet, spicy and resins.

Chypre (F/M)—Sweet, warm, soft notes. These are combinations of resins, citrus and woods. The name is French for the island of Cyprus, birthplace of Venus. Examples include oakmoss, bergamot, labdanum and sandalwood. Miss Dior, Crêpe de Chine and Femme are classic Chypre-type perfumes.

Subgroups: fruity, floral, animal, fresh, green, woody, leathery, coniferous.

Green (M/F)—Fresh and simple, this group includes lavender, pine and mint. Perfumes of this group include Acqua di Selva, English Lavender and Silvestre.

Subgroups: fresh, spicy.

Fougère (M)—Named after the French word for "fern," this group includes lavender, oakmoss and coumarin (tonka bean). Fougere fragrance concepts include Skin Bracer, Kouros, Brut and Boss Sport.

Subgroups: fresh, woody, sweet, floral.

Citrus (M)—One of the oldest fragrance concepts, this group includes all the citrus-fruit peels, petitgrain, neroli, bergamot, Eucalyptus citriodora and lemon thyme. Examples include English Leather, Drakkar and Hermes.

Subgroups: floral, fantasy, fresh, green.

Perfume Notes

Fragrance blending is so analogous to music, we even borrow the terminology. The terms *top, middle* and *base notes* are used to define essential oils based on their evaporation rates, which also reflect their fragrance. Fragrances often described as "light and airy," such as citruses, are considered top notes. Oils we think of as heavy with a tendency to linger, such as patchouli and vetiver, are base notes. Some essential oils are so complex that they fit into more than one category. Rose, for instance, is sometimes categorized as a middle or base note. Peppermint can be described as either a top note or a middle note.

The most carefully developed perfumes represent varying proportions of all three notes. If you like a light, invigorating perfume, choose a predominance of top notes. If you prefer spicy, sensuous blends, go heavy on the base notes. Suggestions for proportions are given in each category below. Your perfume blend should have a full-bodied character; it should not smell thin or sharp. These are guidelines only—feel free to rely on instinct and inspiration, following every spark of creative whimsy.

Top Notes—Sometimes called "head notes" or "peaks," top notes are those essential oils that evaporate quickly. In a blend, they are the very first scents that you smell, and they quickly dissipate. They tend to be light, fresh, sharp or penetrating. The first impression they create lasts no longer than 30 minutes. In perfumery, top notes generally constitute 5-20 percent of the blend.

Therapeutically, many top notes are fast-acting, stimulating, and uplifting to the spirit, making them useful in the treatment of depression. Examples include all the citruses, melissa, and eucalyptus.

Middle Notes—Also called "bouquets," "heart notes" or "modifiers," middle notes create the main body of the blend, rounding it out with soothing, soft tones. The scent of a middle note unfolds anywhere between a few moments to three hours after application. They usually account for 50-80 percent of the blend.

In therapy, middle notes are harmonizing and balancing to both body and mind. Many tend to affect digestion. Middle notes include chamomile, cypress, marjoram, lavender and geranium, as well as seed oils such as dill, celery, fennel, anise and coriander.

Base Notes—Deep, warm and sensuous, base notes help make blends longer-lasting. Their staying power makes them predominate even several hours after application, and they may linger long after the top and middle notes have evaporated.

It takes the proper proportion of a base note to give a blend depth and intensity. When used sparingly and mixed with middle and top notes, most base notes are quite pleasant, but when used alone or allowed to predominate in a formula, they can be overpowering. Base notes are so strong they usually make up only 5 percent of a total blend. Some of the more pleasant base notes, such as sandalwood, cedarwood, frankincense and jasmine, can be used in larger amounts. Base notes include most of the woods, resins and gums, including spikenard, vetiver, myrrh and patchouli.

In therapy, base notes are sedating and can be used to treat anxiety, stress, impatience and insomnia, and to promote relaxation.

Top, Middle and Base Notes

This is by no means a complete list of all the oils, but it will give you some sense of how to categorize them.

* middle-to-base
** top-to-middle

Top Notes	Middle Notes		Base Notes
basil	black pepper	marjoram	benzoin
bergamot	chamomile	neroli*	cedarwood
eucalyptus**	clary sage	petitgrain	frankincense
grapefruit	coriander	pine	jasmine
lemon	cypress*	rose*	myrrh
lemongrass	fennel	rosemary	patchouli
lime	geranium	thyme	rose absolute
mandarin	hyssop	ylang-ylang*	sandalwood
peppermint**	juniper		spikenard
tangerine	lavender		vetiver

Perfume Fixatives

Most fixative oils—including benzoin, balsam of Peru, balsam of tolu, clary sage, orris root, patchouli, sandalwood, vetiver, angelica, frankincense, styrax, oakmoss, and most balsams, gums and oleoresins—are base notes. They have the ability to carry lighter scents and keep them from evaporating too quickly, so the entire blend lasts longer. One nice aspect of fixative oils is that although some are quite expensive, your investment will increase with time as the fragrance improves. Unlike most oils, which must be carefully stored away from heat and oxygen, fixative oils improve with oxidization. We recommend storing fixatives in bottles with lots of air, shaking them often to distribute the oxygen. Fixatives, particularly orris root, are also used to keep the scent of potpourri alive.

Raw patchouli oil, for example, is clear yellow when it is first extracted from the plant. You can almost see through it. Like most fixatives, it turns amber as it ages, finally becoming a deep brown and thickening to a syrupy consistency. The smell also changes, from a harsh scent to a softened, vanilla-like aroma. People often have an aversion to "young" patchouli, but these same people don't even recognize it—and actually often enjoy it—after it has aged for seven years.

Many traditional base notes were once derived from the glands of various animals. Musk (from deer), civet (cat) and castoreum (beavers) were used as fixatives by perfumers. Another animal fixative, ambergris, comes from the intestinal lining of the sperm whale. Although such products once played an important role in the perfume industry, they are for the most part produced synthetically today and are only of interest to the historical-minded aromatherapist.

ASPECTS OF BLENDING

Odor Intensity

Because essential oils vary in odor intensity, we add much smaller amounts of some oils to our blends than others. For example, to obtain equal smell representation in a simple blend of German chamomile and lavender, it would take about five drops of lavender to only one drop of chamomile. Other examples of essential oils with high odor intensities are peppermint, patchouli, spikenard, cinnamon, ylang-ylang, clary sage and jasmine. Keep in mind that all blends change with time, and that different notes become prominent at different times, depending on how long the perfume has aged and whether you are smelling it in the bottle or on the skin. Perfumes also smell different on different people. Biopsychologist Charles Wysocki discovered that body chemistry and skin type play a great role in determining how long a fragrance will last. Molecules in the oils are more easily absorbed and retained by oily skin and act on a time-release principle.

Beginning Blending

The middle notes are the easiest to dive into. If you want to be very safe, choose a middle note that can also be regarded as a base note (see the chart on the preceding page) or add only a tiny amount of a base oil. Then finish the blend with at least one top note.

One trick for beginning blenders is to start with an oil that has a fairly complex chemistry, which will tend to already smell like a blend. Geranium, for example, contains the herby fragrance (geranyl) common to most scented geraniums, a definite rose scent, a pinelike fragrance (isomenthone) and the fragrance of lemon (citronellal), among other constituents. By using geranium you begin with a premixed "blend" of rose, herb, pine and citrus. You can now expand your formula by adding small amounts of other oils, one at a time.

Again, the safest route is to add a second oil that blends well with the complex one. When in doubt, choose the type of fragrance already contained in the complex oil. In the case of geranium, that might be a wood such as cedarwood or sandalwood, a floral such as rose or a citrus—or perhaps bergamot or petitgrain for a more sophisticated fragrance. Finally, add a very small amount of an accent oil to top off the blend. Clary sage, for example, would make for a headier fragrance, and spearmint would liven things up.

One interesting way to expand upon fragrances in a blend is to choose oils that are very similar to each other, such as a combination of peppermint and spearmint, one of lemon and bergamot, or perhaps neroli and another of the citrus group. Most of the spices also make intriguing combinations; try a mix of cinnamon and clove, of ginger and cardamom. Although any of these scents is distinctive on its own, two similar oils mixed together play a confusing and delightful trick on the nose as they play off one another. You can't pinpoint the aroma, which makes it seem complicated and mysterious.

In his standard essential-oil text *Perfumes, Cosmetics and Soaps,* Poucher gives examples of how trace amounts of one oil can change an entire blend. For example, adding a very small quantity of patchouli to a rose base alters the odor very slightly, but makes it smell like a bouquet of white roses instead of red roses (and since patchouli is a fixative, the fragrance is retained much longer).

To sharpen your nose, you can try methods similar to those used by perfumery students. The table we have provided in this chapter of contrasting and similar odors was prepared by the famous perfumer Jean Carles of Grasse, France, known as "Mr. Nose," who was responsible for famous creations such as Tabu, Aqua Brava and Emir. Dissatisfied with the way he had been taught perfume-making—a trial-and-error approach he termed "happy-go-lucky"—Carles developed a systematic study of blending. Each day, the olfactory student compares a series of essential oils to others that are either similar or contrasting. The apprenticeship period takes many years to complete.

According to Charles:

> Anyone may acquire a highly developed sense of smell, as this is merely a matter of practice. A good nose—that is, an excellent olfactory memory—is not enough to produce a good perfumer. By the term "a nose" . . . is meant a perfumer who is able to distinguish a pure product from an adulterated product, who can tell lavender 50 percent from lavender 40 percent. I myself, in spite of my long experience [50 years], am only a beginner in comparison to the old "noses" whom I met at Grasse at the beginning of my career and who were able to detect olfactorily the geographical area [from which] a given oil of neroli or . . . lavender came.

Perfumer Marcel Carles, son of Jean Carles, describes how he learned blending:

> When you smell lemon it contrasts with sandalwood, sandalwood contrasts with cloves, cloves with orange—you are smelling very contrasting odors. It is much easier to memorize the smell of each of these products individually . . . When you have finished the study of odor by contrasts, you start over again with the study of odor by family. But here it is difficult to distinguish lemon from bergamot [or] from tangerine . . . The student whose olfactory memory has been trained in elementary things can go on to the more difficult exercises of studying the odors both by contrast and by family.

Fragrance blends usually improve with age. It takes at least several weeks for a blend to develop its full aroma. During this time, the single essential oils in the blend merge into a cohesive unit. The resulting perfume displays an individual character that is far greater than the sum of its parts.

Therapeutic Blending

Safety

Safety is the most important consideration when choosing ingredients for a blend. It is important to use only high-quality oils, especially for therapeutic applications. Be sure to research the oils you have chosen in order to become familiar with any properties or actions that may not be desirable in a given situation. Review the Safety section in the "Guidelines for Use" chapter.

Purpose

The intended use will help you decide on the most appropriate ingredients for your creation. Consider the condition and symptoms the blend will be used to treat, as well as the subject's state of mind. A blend destined for cosmetic application requires identification of the intended user's skin type (see chapter on "Skin Care").

Application

Decide on the most appropriate method for applying the essential-oil blend. Is it best applied by massage, inhalation, foot bath or some other method? Will your blend be most suitable in a vegetable oil, in alcohol, in water or in some other type of carrier? All of these factors will help you determine the final ingredients and dilution of the blend.

Step-by-Step Blending

Before you begin, take a minute to focus your mind. Take a few deep breaths, relax and center yourself. Think about the purpose of your blend.

Olfactory Study of Essential Oils

Notes	Studies 1	2	3	4	5	6	7	8
Citrus	Lemon	Bergamot	Tangerine	Orange	Orange	Bit Orange	Petigrain	Lime
Woodsy	Sandalwood	Cedar	Vetivert	Patchouly	Oakmoss	Oakmoss	Pine	Cypress
Spicy	Cloves	Cinnamon	Pimento	Nutmeg	Pepper	Pimento	Juniper	Coriander
Anise	Anise	Badine	Fennel	Fennel	Basil	Tarragon	Cumin	Caraway
Rose	Absolute	—	—	Bulgarian	Geranium	Geranium	Geranium	Palmarosa
Rustic *(Camphor-Like)*	Lavender	Lavendin	Span. Lav.	Rosemary	Thyme	Eucalyptus	Bay	Myrtle/Sage
Balsam	Bal. Peru	Bal. Tolu	Vanilla	Tonka	Styrax	Labdanum	Clary Sage	Bal Copaiba
Floral *(Absolutes)*	Jasmine	Tuberose	Jonquil	Hyacinth	Narcissus	Violet	Cassie	Orris
Resin	Frank.	Benzoin	Opopanax	Myrrh	Elemi	Galbanum	—	—
Orange/ Citronella	Citronella	Lemongrass	Verbena	Melissa	Neroli	Petitgrain	—	—
Mint & Misc.	Peppermint	Spearmint	Pennyroyal	Marjoram	Rosewood	—	Winter.	Cajeput

This chart, prepared by Perfumer Jean Carles for his students, has been simplified for your use. Read across the line for oils with similar scents. Read down the column for contrasting oils. Combining both similar and contrasting oils are used as blending techniques. Carles had his students spend at least a day studying just one line or column to become more familiar with the art of scent blending.

Keep detailed notes of your experiments, including your failures. This is very important. You can lose a successful blend forever if you don't write it down. Be sure to label each blend with the date, ingredients, dilution, name of the blend, and any other useful information.

To begin creating your blend, make a list of all the oils that are appropriate or desirable for your particular purposes. If you are a beginner, it is best to restrict the list to five oils or less. Smell the oils one by one and try to imagine how they will blend with one another. Remember that many oils are overpowering when smelled directly from the bottle. Wave the cap briefly under your nose for a better appreciation of the true fragrance.

Once you have sampled each oil individually, determine how well they combine. You can hold the bottle caps to your nose in different combinations or, better yet, use strips of blotter paper labeled with the names of the different oils. Place a dab of oil on each strip and wave them together in different combinations.

Required Supplies

Blotter paper
Clean, empty bottles
Essential oils
Carriers: oils, glycerin, distilled water, hydrosol, alcohol
Funnel (optional)
Eyedropper(s)
Cleanup supplies: paper towels, tissues, alcohol
Labels, pencil, notebook

Now you are ready to mix. Start with small proportions, blending drop by drop. Sniff as you go, and continue to make notes on how the blend progresses. It is easiest to mix essential oils together before adding them to the carrier.

When you are satisfied with your blend, add it to a carrier or base such as oil, alcohol, hydrosol, water or even vinegar. If you prefer, you may leave your blends in concentrated form. They will be much more versatile, lending themselves to a variety of applications.

Sample Recipes

Here are a few ideas to get you started. All of the following recipes may be diluted in 1 ounce of carrier oil (a 2-percent dilution) to make a massage or body oil, or in an equal amount of jojoba for a perfume. As an exercise, start by adding one drop of each oil. Sniff as you add each drop, and observe how it changes the blend. If you feel adventurous, alter the proportions to suit yourself.

In order not to contaminate each essential oil with the one you used before it, use separate droppers, or rinse your dropper in vodka or pure grain alcohol between oils and dry it before dipping it into the next scent. This way you won't need a different dropper for each scent.

Afternoon Delight

4 drops orange
2 drops geranium
3 drops lavender
4 drops sandalwood

Adolescent Airs

5 drops lavender
4 drops mandarin
2 drops neroli
2 drops vanilla

Earth Dew

4 drops juniper
3 drops cedarwood
2 drops frankincense
3 drops jasmine

Floral Spice

2 drops ylang-ylang
2 drops vetiver
6 drops bergamot
3 drops cardamom

Kiss-Me-Quick

2 drops rose
3 drops jasmine
6 drops grapefruit
2 drops ylang-ylang

Energy

2 drops black pepper
6 drops lemon
3 drops rosemary
1 drop peppermint

Perfume/Cologne

A perfume contains more essential oils and a higher percentage of alcohol than a cologne. Colognes were originally designed for splashing rather than dabbing. Because natural perfumes are much more concentrated, they command a higher price. As a carrier for either perfume or cologne, you can use vodka or pure grain alcohol diluted with distilled water. Nevada, Oregon and Alaska sell 94-percent alcohol to the public. If you prefer an oil base, consider the application and refer to the section on carrier oils in the "Guidelines for Use" chapter. Jojoba is best.

Alcohol Concentrations

Product	Percent Alcohol
Extrait or perfume	5-30%
Parfûm de toilette or Eau de parfum	8-15%
Eau de toilette	4-8%
Eau de cologne	3-5%
Splash cologne	1-3%

You are now ready to start creating your own ultimate perfume!

Ancient Perfume Formulations

Chemist Giuseppe Conato, former director of the Laboratory of Experimental Archaeology at Italy's National Research Council, studies ancient perfumes. In the 1970s, he journeyed to the Black Sea to investigate Cleopatra's ancient perfume factory near the En-Gedi oasis. The factory, now partially reconstructed, has two drying kilns, revolving grinding mills for herbs, two large tubs to macerate herbs with oil, a stove to prepare ointments, and a waiting room complete with stone seats. A tower once stood there, possibly to view the plantations of fragrant plants that surrounded the factory.

More accurately, we might call this a cosmetic factory. Perfumes of that era were vegetable-based body oils made by grinding dried herbs and soaking them in hot oil. Then the oil was pressed, either through a bag (Egyptian-style) or with a screw press

Natural Ingredients in Commercial Perfumes

Here are a few examples of natural ingredients in some popular commercial perfumes of today. This is by no means a complete list of ingredients; synthetics are also used in each blend.

For Men:

Calvin

Top notes:	lavender, anise, bergamot, petitgrain, lemon
Middle notes:	geranium, marjoram, clary sage, rose, juniper
Base notes:	patchouli, vetiver, sandalwood, oakmoss

Obsession

Top notes:	bergamot, lemon, clary sage
Middle notes:	rosewood, cinnamon
Base notes:	cedarwood, patchouli, sandalwood, benzoin, vanilla

Brut

Top notes:	lavender, anise, lemon, basil, bergamot
Middle notes:	geranium, ylang-ylang, jasmine
Base notes:	sandalwood, vetiver, patchouli, oakmoss, vanilla, tonka

Boss

Top notes:	bergamot, lemon, mandarin, artemisia
Middle notes:	juniper, clary sage, mace, geranium, jasmine, rose
Base notes:	patchouli, cedar, sandalwood, tonka

Old Spice

Top notes:	orange, lemon, anise, clary sage
Middle notes:	cinnamon, geranium, jasmine, pimento berry
Base notes:	vanilla, cedarwood, frankincense, benzoin

For Women:

Tabu

Top notes:	orange, neroli, bergamot, coriander
Middle notes:	ylang-ylang, jasmine, clove, rose
Base notes:	vetiver, cedarwood, patchouli, benzoin, sandalwood

Shalimar

Top notes:	lemon, bergamot, mandarin, rosewood
Middle notes:	rose, jasmine, orris
Base notes:	vanilla, benzoin, patchouli, vetiver

Chanel No. 5

Top notes:	bergamot, lemon, neroli
Middle notes:	jasmine, rose, orris, ylang-ylang
Base notes:	vetiver, sandalwood, cedar, vanilla

White Shoulders

Top notes:	neroli, bergamot
Middle notes:	jasmine, rose, tuberose, clove, orris
Base notes:	sandalwood, benzoin

Anais Anais

Top notes:	neroli, galbanum
Middle notes:	jasmine, rose, tuberose, orris, ylang-ylang
Base notes:	sandalwood, cedar, vetiver

Perfume Formulas Throughout History

1800 B.C. Babylon
- Cedar, myrrh, cypress
- Labdanum, Myrrh, Storax

1300 B.C. Egypt
- *Kyphi* (Tutankhamen)—calamus, mastic, henna, juniper, spikenard

1200 B.C. Egypt
- "Anointing Oil" (Moses)—Myrrh (4 parts), cinnamon (2 parts), calamus (2 parts), olive oil
- Frankincense, myrrh, cinnamon, cassia, cyperus, saffron, terebinth (pistachio)
- Styrax, labanum, galbanum, frankincense, myrrh, cinnamon, cassia, honey, raisins
- Onycha, galbanum, myrrh, frankincense, spices

600 B.C. Greece
- "Megaleion"—Burnt resin, cassia, cinnamon, myrrh

100 B.C. Rome
- "Telinum" (Caesar)—Fenugreek, cyperus, calamus, melilot, marjoram, honey, maro, onphacium
- "Rhodinum"—Rose, crocus, cinnamon, calamus, honey, rush, salt, alkanet, wine, onphacium
- "Myrtum Lurum" (Oil of Persia)—Marjoram, lily, fenugreek, myrrh, cassia, spikenard, rush, cinnamon, myrtle, bay, onphacium
- "Metopium"—Bitter almond, cardamom, rush, calamus, honey, myrrh, balsam, turpentine resin, onphacium
- "Regale Unguentum" (aphrodisiac for the kings of Parthia)—Costus, cinnamon, cardamom, lavender, myrrh, clover, cassia, styrax, labdanum, balsam, calamus, rush, bay, cassia, cyperus, saffron, henna, marjoram, lotus, honey, wine, onphacium
- "Cyprinum"—Cyperus, cardamom, calamus, wormwood, onphacium
- "Telinum"—Cyperus, calamus, melilot, fenugreek, marjoram, honey, onphacium

A.D 100 Rome
- "Amarakinon" (Pliny)—Spikenard, myrrh, cinnamon, costus
- "Susinon"—Lily, balsam, cinnamon, saffron, myrrh, onphacium (some versions include calamus, cardamom, honey)

1100 India
- Jasmine, cardamom, pine, cloves, coriander, basil, sesame oil
- Costus, pandanus, agarwood, chamac

1100 China
- Rose, camphor, cassia, citrus
- Rose, camphor, cassia, citrus, herbs, alcohol

1200 Europe
- "Queen of Hungary Waters"—Rosemary, lavender
- "Carmelite Water"—Melissa, angelica, herbs

1500 England (Queen Elizabeth)
- Musk, rose water, sugar
- Marjoram, benzoin in rose water

1600 Europe
- "Casting Water"—Herbs, rose water

1700 France
- "Brown Windsor Soap"—Bergamot, cloves, lavender
- "Eau De Cologne" (Farina)—Neroli, bergamot, lavender, rosemary, rectified grape wine
- Louis XIV's favorite—Aloewood, nutmeg, cloves, storax, benzoin, rosewater
- "Poudre a La Maréchale"—Ambrette, cloves, coustadon, calamus, iris, dill, lemon peel, neroli, ambergris

1800
- "Jicky" (Guerlain)—Bergamot, orris, lavender, synthetics

1900
- "La Rose Jacqueminot" (Coty)—Rose, violet
- "Chypre" (Coty)—Citrus, bergamot, sandalwood, gum resins

1920
- "Emeraude" (Coty)—Spices, resins
- "L'Origan" (Coty)—Marjoram
- "L'Heure Bleue" —Resin, labdanum, balsam of Peru, synthetics
- "Numero Cinque" (Chanel) Chanel No. 5—Ylang-ylang, jasmine, rose, animal scents, aldehyde
- "Shalimar" (Guerlain)—Sandalwood, amber, bergamot, musk, civet
- "My Sin" (Lanvin)—Florals, synthetics
- "Arpége" (Lanvin)—Jasmine, floral scents

1930
- "Tabu" (Dana)—Patchouli, oakmoss, musk, bergamot, neroli, ylang-ylang
- "Joy" (Patou)—Bulgarian Rose, jasmine, synthetics
- "Shocking" (Schiaparelli)—Patchouli, synthetic hyacinth

1940
- "Miss Dior" (Dior)—Patchouli, citrus, sandalwood

1950
- "Youth Dew" (Estée Lauder)—Frankincense, patchouli, vetiver, clove, musk
- "Cabochard" (Grés)— Spices

1970
- "Aramis 700"—Patchouli
- "Bill Blass" (Bill Blass)—Patchouli
- "Charlie" (Revlon)—Synthetics
- "Opium" (St. Laurent)—Incense resins, spices, florals

1980
- "Andron" (Jovan)—Androsterone

(Greek method). The oil base was often *onphacium*, an almost odorless oil pressed from unripe olives. It had only a faint herblike scent and contained so little fat that it spread easily over the skin without being greasy.

Another ingredient employed in the factory was Dead Sea salt, which contains an unusually high concentration of mineral salts (magnesium, potassium, and sodium chlorides)—ten times more than open sea salt. Another component was the famous Black Sea mud, called *asphaltite* by Pliny. Extracted from mud that was rich in petroleum deposits, this "pitch of Judea" was used in a popular beauty treatment for the skin.

Blending with Imagination

Edmond Roudnitska, perfumer for the House of Dior and Rochas, carries 40 years of recipes in one small spiral notebook. He creates not with his nose but with imagination. To explain his olfactory genius, Roudnitska says:

> A thought comes to mind. I foresee, I visualize a certain form for a perfume . . . I try first to outline or sketch out the form with products that are most familiar to me, and then I try to modify it, and, step by step, this study goes along, because a study of this nature can last several years, and as it does, I might have my hand on some new raw material, and I say to myself, "Well, now, this might be just the thing I need to complete the form." To create a perfume, you have to live entirely in the universe of odor, think in that universe and, being in it, visualize forms—it is very abstract.

Just as the chef starts in the kitchen, the perfumer starts in the laboratory of a perfumery by studying the odors, smelling one after the other. When he has practiced this a great deal, he begins to make small experiments and learns to combine the odors, as a *chef de cuisine* makes different combinations of tastes, or as a painter makes combinations of colors. It's never done the same way twice.

12

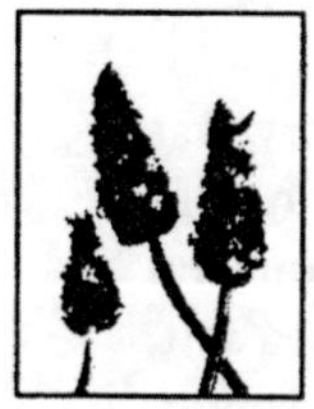

Extracting Essential Oils

Ever since it was discovered that fragrance could be isolated from plants, human beings have experimented with the best way to accomplish this. Much has been learned since the time that plants were first added to animal fats or steeped in water to extract their fragrances, and refinements in techniques are still being sought today. The goal for the alchemists of the second and third centuries AD was to capture the "quintessence" of the plant—hence "essential" oils, describing the "soul" or "spirit" of the plant.

DISTILLATION

The distillation process of extracting essential oils utilizes steam, heat and condensation. About 80 percent of all natural oils produced are extracted by distillation. For hundreds of years it has been the best method of extracting pure essential oils, and even with the myriad of techniques available today, it still provides a very pure product.

During distillation fragrant plants exposed to boiling water or steam release their essential oils through evaporation. The oil-laden steam rises and enters narrow tubing that is cooled by an outside source: a larger vessel surrounding the tubing contains cold water that circulates constantly to keep it cold. The tubing is designed (often in a lengthy spiral) to provide a lot of surface area so that the steam, which contains both essential-oil gases and water vapor, will cool as quickly as possible, thus creating condensation (little droplets of water). As the steam turns back into water and essential oil, both are collected in a vessel traditionally called the "Florentine flask" (named for a city known for essential-oil distillation during the Renaissance). Because oil and water don't mix, the essential oil floats on top of the water and can be separated easily. (Some exceptions are oil of clove, birch, wintergreen and anise, which sink to the bottom of the water.) A sophisticated distiller will separate the essential oil into one vial and the water (called "*hydrosol*") into another. Otherwise, the oil must be siphoned or skimmed off.

Examples of commonly distilled plants are lavender, geranium, rosemary and eucalyptus. In general, plants are distilled when they are fresh. Dense or thick plant material, especially roots and seeds, are crushed or chopped before distillation for more efficient extraction of the essential oil. The technical term for this process is "comminution." Comminution is not necessary with very delicate plant parts, such as leaves and flowers, because the steam penetrates them easily.

The amount of essential oil produced depends on four main criteria: the length of distillation time, the temperature, the operating pressure and, most importantly, the type and quality of the plant material. Other details that affect yield are harvest time (time of day as well as time of year), climatic conditions and the amount of volatile oil each plant produces. Typically, the yield of essential oils in plants is between 0.005 and 10 percent. For example, plants that produce a relatively high percentage of essential oils, such as sage, thyme and rosemary, take approximately 500 pounds of plant material to produce 32 ounces of essential oil. These factors affect the price of the oil.

Historically, there have been three types of distillation: water distillation, water-steam distillation and steam distillation. Water distillation is sometimes referred to as "indirect" steam distillation. In this method, plant material is soaked in water and heated until it boils. The resulting steam from the boiling water carries the volatile oils with it. Cooling and condensation subsequently separate the oil from the water. This method requires very little equipment and can be done on the spot immediately after harvesting, making it quite inexpensive. Apart from its slowness, the disadvantage of this technique is that both materials and scent deteriorate from constant heat exposure.

The second method utilizes steam. In this more sophisticated method, the leafy plant material is placed on a grill above the hot water, and the steam passes through the plant material. The leaves must be carefully distributed on the grill to allow for even steaming and thorough extraction.

The third technique, sometimes referred to as "direct" steam distillation, is the most common for essential-oil extraction. In this process, no water is placed inside the distillation tank itself. Instead, steam is directed into the tank from an outside source. The essential oils are released from the plant material when the steam bursts the sacs that contain the tiny molecules of oil. Again, at this stage the process of condensation and separation is standard. Direct steam distillation is quick, causing minimal deterioration of delicate essential-oil components, and produces a higher quality essential oil than do the water and water-steam distillation methods.

As popular and well established as distillation is, there still are several drawbacks. One is that steam, especially when it enters plant material from the bottom, does not always disperse evenly. As a result, distillation takes a longer time and extraction can be inefficient. In addition, the heating and cooling needed for distillation require a lot of energy. Steam must be created with fire, which burns a lot of wood, or with gas or electricity, which can be expensive. Refrigeration to cool down the steam is also costly. In addition, as many as 48 hours may be required to thoroughly distill a plant. Over such a long period of time, oxidation may occur which chemically alters the original makeup of the essential oil, often with undesirable results. Some of the problems of steam distillation have been remedied by the invention of other extraction methods, discussed later in this section.

Improved Distillation Techniques

Many flowers are so fragile that exposure to the high heat of steam distillation destroys their delicate scents. The new extraction methods still utilize steam, but the techniques have improved. Thanks to a shorter processing time and lower temperature, a superior product results. New energy-efficient methods also help to cut costs.

Turbo Distillation

Hard plant materials such as roots, seeds and barks are processed by turbo distillation. Steaming is combined with cohobation—a process in which the water, known as the "hydrolate," is recycled back into the still to produce more steam. The plant material is soaked and softened, then continuously agitated as it is exposed to the recycled steam. This can reduce the processing time by half.

Hydrodiffusion

In hydrodiffusion, a more energy-efficient variation of direct steam distillation, the steam is forced through the plant material from the top, rather than the bottom, of the still. This method is much gentler than those described above, and because less time is required for distillation, the resulting essential oil comes closer to the true scent of the plant. Hydrodiffusion is used only with fresh leafy herbs; roots and seeds are left to other, more efficient forms of distillation.

Vacuum Distillation

Vacuum distillation is a very sophisticated technique in which the steam never comes in contact with the plant material. Unlike many other methods, the vacuum process provides "dry" distillation, where the steam does not enter the still itself. Instead, the steam is contained in a heating jacket outside the still, somewhat like a double boiler. A vacuum effect within the still releases the essential oil from the plant material at a lower temperature. The oil can be collected whole for use in aromatherapy, or portions of the distillate can be collected as they emerge from the condenser.

Fractioning

Fractioning is a technique used to separate specific chemical components from the whole oil. Because each aromatic component in a plant has its own boiling point, each evaporates at a different rate. It is therefore possible to separate the components as they emerge from the condenser, isolating and eliminating individual components as desired. This option is more useful to a perfumer who wants to boost or eliminate a distinctive scent, or to a chemist who wants to adulterate an oil by increasing a specific aromatic component, than it is to an aromatherapist concerned with developing a natural product.

Continuous Distillation

Continuous distillation, a new process recently introduced in France, utilizes discarded tree branches such as juniper, eucalyptus and pine, which are cut into small pieces for distillation and exposed to repeated steaming. One method, described by Marcel Lavabre, a former distiller and present owner of Aroma Vera, involves continuous feeding of plant material through a tube in which it is exposed to steam. As fresh plant material enters the tube, exhausted plant material is pushed out the other end. The plant material receives extensive exposure to the steam, greatly reducing distillation time. This method also allows for fractionation of different constituents.

Molecular Distillation

Also known as rectifying, redistilling involves distilling an oil two and sometimes three times. This process eliminates the heavier parts of the essential oil, making it smell more the way it does in nature. Some situations, however, require the use of the raw oil produced during the first distillation. In the case of peppermint, the heavier parts contained in the oil from the initial distillation are "hotter," so this oil is a good choice for use as a liniment. The lighter, redistilled oil is usually preferred for flavoring or for its emotional impact. A number of oils can be redistilled with excellent results, including camphor and eucalyptus. The extraction process is rarely indicated on the label, so it may be difficult to tell if you are getting a redistilled oil—unless you have a trained nose or a whole oil which to compare against it.

OTHER METHODS OF EXTRACTION

Plants are also extracted by methods other than distillation. These include cold expression, enfleurage, solvent extraction and carbon-dioxide extraction.

Cold Expression

Cold expression is sometimes referred to as "scarification." This method of extraction is used for citrus fruits, which contain essential oil-bearing pouches in their peels. The peel is shredded, then mechanically pressed. The resulting emulsion, consisting of essential oil, juice, water and fruit particles, is either filtered or passed through a clarifying centrifuge. The essential oil, which floats on top, is then separated out.

Natural plant waxes resulting from cold expression may contribute to a slight cloudiness or create some sediment in the final oil. This usually does not present a problem unless it is important for the oil to be visually clear, or if it will be used in a diffuser that may be clogged by the sediment. The sediment can be removed by filtering the oil through a fine cloth or a paper filter.

Citrus skins are not always pressed. For instance, lemon and lime peel are also distilled. The smell of the resulting oil is more reminiscent of candy than the fresh-peel smell of cold-pressed citrus oils. Distilled oil of lime is used in many soft drinks, including Coca-Cola, 7-Up and Pepsi. Oils produced in this way are considered inferior apart from one advantage: they may not be as photosensitive as most expressed citrus oils. Unfortunately, the citrus industry often uses chemicals and pesticides that are sprayed directly on the peel and carry over to the essential oil when the peel is pressed. Distilled citrus oils are less likely to contain these pesticide residues. Buy pressed citrus essential oil extracted from organically grown fruit whenever possible.

Enfleurage

Virtually obsolete today, enfleurage is perhaps the oldest method of extracting fragrance from plants. It is used for delicate plants that are unable to withstand the high heat of distillation, or for those that continue to exude fragrance after they are picked, such as tuberose and jasmine. Refined lard and tallow are still used in enfleurage today, as they have been for centuries. With their excellent ability to pick up fragrance molecules from flowers, animal fats are the preferred medium for this type of extraction.

In the traditional enfleurage process, fat is spread thickly on plates of glass and covered with freshly picked flowers. The layers of glass are sealed to retain the scent. The flowers are left undisturbed for 24 to 48 hours, then replaced with fresh ones. This time-consuming, labor-intensive process is repeated for several weeks until the fat is saturated with the fragrance of the flowers. Then the fat is gently warmed and filtered. The resulting product is called a *pomade*. In ages past, pomade was used directly on the skin and hair. Today, it is usually "washed" with alcohol to remove the fat. The alcohol carries the essential oil and is separated from the fat by chilling. At this stage, the product is called an *extrait*.

An *absolute d'enfleurage* is created in the next stage of processing. This semisolid product is made by distilling off the alcohol. The final product is coded with a number that represents the number of times fresh flowers were placed on the fat. If you find a "jasmine #42," for example, it means the flowers were replaced 42 times. The higher the number, the finer (and generally more expensive) the absolute. Technically, absolutes—used mainly by the perfume industry—are not essential oils, though they contain them.

An inferior by-product called *absolute de chassis* is made from the flowers after they have been removed from the fat. Whatever essential oils are left in the blossoms are extracted with solvents. The perfume industry uses the resulting oil to add fullness to synthetic jasmine compounds.

To make your own infused jasmine oil at home, use almond oil as a substitute for animal fat. See the "Guidelines for Use" chapter for directions.

Solvent Extraction

Solvent extraction has made it possible to create a whole range of oils that could never be produced before because their structures are too delicate to withstand other methods of extraction. This is because solvents do not require high heat and water for extraction. However, the method is not without drawbacks and controversy.

Solvents used for extraction include petroleum ether, hexane, toluene, butane, methane, propane, as well as the more toxic, even carcinogenic solvents benzene and acetone. The plant material is submerged in and agitated with the solvent which dissolves the volatile oils—as well as the waxes and pigments—in the plant. The solvent is removed through evaporation under pressure. The result is a sticky, soft wax called a *concrete*. Because of the waxes and pigments it contains, the product may have cosmetic applications while still in the concrete stage. To continue the extraction process, the concrete is mixed with ethyl alcohol and chilled so the solidified waxes can be filtered out, leaving essential oils diluted in alcohol. The last step is to remove the alcohol by vacuum-distilling the mixture. The final product is called an *absolute*.

Absolutes are said to be relatively free of the solvents and alcohol used during extraction, but solvent-extracted oils, especially those extracted with hexane, may retain a slight residue in the final product. The least harmful solvents are butane, propane and methane, but one can never be sure what was used. Because solvents are sometimes odorless, it may be difficult to detect them. Solvent-extracted oils should never be taken orally or used to flavor food. Because solvent residues may be present, absolutes are not generally recommended for use in aromatherapy, but are suitable for creating natural perfumes. However, new methods of extracting essential oils are being developed which are said to remove all of the solvents.

A *resinoid* is another product derived through solvent or alcohol extraction. The main distinction between resinoids and concretes is that resinoids are produced from plant matter such as tree saps and exudates (such as frankincense, mastic, labdanum, tolu and the lichen oakmoss), whereas concretes are extracted from fresh plant matter.

Carbon-Dioxide Extraction

Supercritical carbon-dioxide (CO_2) extraction is a relatively new process used to obtain essential oils through high pressure and low heat. CO_2 extraction is an aromatherapist's dream come true for several reasons. The extraction takes place in a closed chamber and is completed within minutes, so even the most volatile and heat-sensitive fragrance compounds can be collected undamaged and without solvent residues, retaining both fragrance quality and physiological activity. Because the solvent CO_2 is a gas, it is easily—and totally—removed when the pressure is released.

CO_2 extracts come close to the flavor and aroma of the plant, making them excellent candidates for food flavorings, and today the process is used extensively for this purpose. (Although distillation results in a pure product, it does not always provide an exact representation of a plant's smell or taste.)

There are two types of CO_2 extraction. The first type produces *selective extracts*, obtained at a relatively low pressure of 100 pounds per square inch. They are similar (but superior) to distilled products in that they consist almost completely of volatile compounds and usually have a liquid consistency. They are suitable for all aromatherapy applications and perfumery. Examples are ambrette seed, frankincense, myrrh, orris root, black currant and chamomile. The second type of CO_2 extraction produces *total extracts*, which are obtained at considerably higher pressure (350 pounds per square inch). These extracts contain not only essential oils (volatile compounds), but also fats, waxes and plant pigments. This method of extraction is especially useful with plants specific for skin care. It thoroughly extracts all the healing constituents (carotenoids, flavonoids and essential oils), producing a thick orange tar. The application of this technique to extract lipids such as GLA (gamma-linoleic acids) for the cosmetic and health industries holds a great deal of promise. Some examples of total extracts available today are carrot (root), chamomile, ginger, sea buckthorn, coriander, juniper, lovage, rosemary and vanilla. Like selective extracts, totals are used in the food and cosmetics industries, and are also suitable for all aromatherapy applications. Some CO_2 total extracts, such as hops and saw palmetto, are also used in the herb industry.

Until recently, CO_2 extracts were rarely available to the consumer. Today, they are generally more expensive than distilled oils because the equipment investment is high; prices should decrease as demand increases.

QUALITY AND PURITY

Quality and purity are often regarded as the same thing, but there are subtle differences. "Purity" refers to authenticity, the promise that a product is unadulterated. "Quality" is related to the "grade" of an oil, which can be influenced by the growing, processing or extraction methods. These are important concerns for consumers of essential oils, and rightly so. Everyone would like to obtain the best-quality product for the best price. Because most essential oils are produced outside the United States, however, it is sometimes hard to confirm both quality and purity, especially as the growing interest in herb products and essential oils has created levels of demand that are becoming increasingly difficult to meet. This is one reason that many perfume and cosmetics manufacturers have switched to synthetics. Other factors include consistency of aroma and lower cost.

Quality and purity should be especially important to companies or stores that claim to carry "aromatherapy-grade" products. Often store clerks will tell you a line of essential oils is "natural," even when it is synthetic. Like many people, they assume that anything labeled "essential oil" is natural and pure. Unfortunately, this is not always so. Most fragrances used in skin-care products are synthetic, even those found in natural-food stores. It is no secret that rose is the most popular fragrance, but few companies can afford to use the pure oil and still manage to offer their products at a price most consumers can afford.

Because the aromatherapy industry is unregulated by government, self-regulation is vital—although some standards do exist for essential oils sold in pharmacies, or for those that carry a Food Chemical Codex (FCC) rating, a government standard set by the Food and Drug Administration (FDA). Essential oils that carry an FCC rating are food-grade essential oils approved for use as food flavorings or additives; essential oils labeled "USP grade," often available at pharmacies, meet guidelines set by the official *United States Pharmacopoeia*. Still, while such labels may verify the percentage of constituents or which extraction process produced it, neither FCC coding oils nor USP grading guarantee quality.

So how can you be sure you have a good-quality essential oil product? As noted, labeling does not always ensure purity—but it can be an indicator. Ideally, the label should say "pure plant essential oil"; terms such as "fragrance oil" or "perfume oil" typically refer to synthetics, which should not be used for therapeutic aromatherapy application. As an informed consumer, you have tremendous power in the marketplace. Ask your suppliers for all the information they have concerning their products. Insist on purity and integrity in the products you choose. It is helpful if the label and accompanying literature indicate the botanical name of the plant, what part of the plant was used and the country of origin. Many reputable sellers of pure essential oils do not list this information on their labels, but they are usually willing to answer questions.

Adulteration of Essential Oils

Governments may set guidelines for the levels of chemical constituents that an oil should contain, but nature does not always cooperate by remaining consistent from year to year. Unfortunately, unscrupulous vendors try to meet these standards by adding synthetics to their essential oils. Rare and expensive oils are the most likely candidates for adulteration, usually by a seller wanting to increase his margin of profit on the product. It is often difficult for an untrained nose to tell the difference between the very expensive pure essential oils of lemon verbena or melissa, and those mixed with cheap lemongrass or citronella. (In fact, these oils are so often mixed with less expensive oils that you may never have smelled the real thing.)

Another common method of adulterating essential oils is by "extending" (i.e., diluting) them with vegetable oil, alcohol or solvent. One way to check for adulteration with vegetable oil is to put a small drop of the essential oil on a piece of paper. Because they are volatile, most essential oils should evaporate rather quickly, leaving no residue. If an oily stain remains, you should suspect the product has been diluted. The only pure essential oils that leave slight color stains are dark oils such as benzoin and patchouli, the bright blue oils such as German chamomile, and viscous oils such as sandalwood and vetiver. Oils diluted with alcohol can be detected by a slight odor, but it can be hard to tell whether an oil has been diluted with a clear, nonoily, odorless solvent. This is a potentially dangerous situation, because such solvents are readily absorbed into the body when rubbed on the skin or inhaled into the lungs.

Reconstruction of Oils

Pure essential oils can be "reconstructed" by combining specific chemical constituents to match the composition of the natural oil. The constituents may be from natural sources, such as pine or some other easily manipulated oil. Fractioning of essential oils allows for reconstruction from natural sources. A reconstructed rosemary is often created with 20 to 35 natural compounds from other plants that match the main aromatic compounds normally found in real rosemary oil. Rose oil is often extended with the natural compound geraniol (found in geranium and other plants), which has a distinctive roselike scent.

Such adulterations, even if they are from natural sources, are not suitable for aromatherapy. Pure essential oils are thought to contain many aromatic molecules that have not yet been detected—unidentified constituents that are active, integral parts of the whole essential oil. When essential oils are reconstructed, even from natural sources, such trace elements may be missing.

In the future, expensive essential oils such as rose and jasmine may be produced in laboratories. Scientists are experimenting with isolating the cells that produce the oils, then growing them in a soaplike solution. They hope the cultured cells will continue to produce essential oils, just as they do in nature. This process will most probably yield oils suitable for the perfume industry, leaving more of the natural oils for aromatherapy.

Synthetics

Synthetic aromas are not extracted, but are chemically manufactured from a variety of easily manipulated base ingredients, from pine oil to petroleum. Synthetic oils became popular in the 1930s and gained dominance in the cosmetics and body-care industry.

Aromatherapists do not use synthetics, because at best they can only duplicate scent, and most cannot do that well. A number of other problems make synthetics unsuitable for use in aromatherapy. To match a real essential oil as closely as possible, the potent aromatic chemicals used in synthetics must be extended in a solvent base. These potentially toxic solvents may be absorbed through the skin. Perhaps most importantly, there is no substitute for the "life force" in plants grown in the earth and nourished by the sun, rain and other elements.

GETTING IT RIGHT

Until your nose develops aromatherapy savvy, here are some tips to remember:

- Many oils are not produced naturally, so if you see lily of the valley, lotus, magnolia, apricot, coconut, peach, amber, strawberry, hibiscus or apple (and possibly carnation and violet, unless they are very expensive), they are synthetics. In fact, if these particular oils are all of the same brand and are sold with oils you think are natural, be suspicious of the entire selection.
- Use the prices of the very expensive natural extracts of jasmine and rose as a yardstick against which to compare questionable oils. If you find jasmine or rose oil priced significantly lower than $250 per quarter-ounce bottle, or less than $20 per milliliter retail, the oil is probably synthetic (or at best, highly diluted).
- Because you cannot always trust what a label or a store clerk tells you, the best indicator of quality is ultimately your own nose. Becoming a good judge of quality really isn't that difficult. When we bring samples of high-quality oils and synthetics to our aromatherapy classes for students to compare, most are able to pick out the synthetics right away.
- Some companies supply gas chromatographs (GC's) that identify and qualify the proportions and various constituents of the essential oil. However, few consumers are trained to interpret these. Therefore, knowing your source, trusting your supplier and training your nose are probably the best means of monitoring quality.

13

Chemistry of Essential Oils

A good grasp of the basics of essential-oil chemistry can add a new dimension to your aromatherapy skills. Becoming familiar with the actions of chemical constituents will help you use essential oils more effectively because you will better understand why and how they work. The approach to aromatic chemistry explained here was first introduced to students of aromatherapy in France by Daniel Penoel, M.D., and researcher Pierre Franchomme. It was subsequently introduced to a wider audience in the United States by chemist and educator Kurt Schnaubelt, Ph.D.

HOW PLANTS MANUFACTURE ESSENTIAL OILS

Before we delve into the chemistry of essential oils, let's take a look at how they are manufactured within the plant itself. Essential oils are created and stored in specialized plant structures such as secretory cells, glands, glandular hairs, and oil or resin ducts, and they are always segregated from other plant tissues within these areas. The secretory cells that produce the volatile oils trap the photoelectromagnetic energy of the sun and, with the help of glucose, convert it into biochemical energy in the form of aromatic molecules. In a process similar to photosynthesis, plants create essential oils by trapping and transmuting light and energy.

Volatile oils are produced in various parts of plants. For instance, they are found in fruit peels (all citrus), gums and resins (frankincense and myrrh), flowers (rose and lavender), leaves (sage, lemon balm, geranium and peppermint), barks (cinnamon and sassafras), roots (vetiver and valerian), grasses (lemongrass and palmarosa), rhizomes (ginger) and seeds (fennel, anise, cumin, celery, dill and coriander). The citrus species *Citrus bigaradia*, commonly known as bitter orange, provides three different essential oils: petitgrain from the leaf, neroli from the blossom, and bitter orange from the fruit peel.

Plants that produce essential oils do so for a number of reasons critical to their survival. Volatile oils in fragrant flowers attract insects for pollination and reproduction. Some essential oils protect against predators and act as antibacterial agents as the essential oils evaporate from the surface of the leaves. And in times of metabolic disruption, such as a drought, essential oils serve as protection for the plant.

Whole Plants vs. Essential Oils

When we distill the essential oil from a plant, the only therapeutic properties we obtain are those of the volatile oil. Molecules of glycosides and many other plant constituents, such as tannins, saponins and alkaloids, are too large and heavy to carry over in distillation. When you are researching essential oils in an herb book, keep in mind that the properties attributed to the herb do not necessarily apply to the essential oil, but may be related to constituents found only in the whole plant.

Many of the 400,000 to 500,000 known plant species in the world have not yet been tested for essential oils or oil components. Although many plants are thought to produce essential oils or essential-oil components to some degree, the amounts may be undetectable or too minute to extract. In addition, although some plants produce minute to acceptable amounts of essential oils, the sheer quantity of plant material required for commercial production prohibits their use.

Echinacea is a good example. This popular immune-modulating and infection-fighting herb produces trace amounts of volatile oils, but not enough to make essential-oil extraction commercially viable or ecologically sound. On the other hand, some herbs high in volatile oils are not exploited commercially. Osha, for example, is an oil-rich herb valued for its antimicrobial and expectorant properties. We have distilled it at home and found that it yields a good quantity of essential oil. Thus it seems that the essential-oil properties of osha and many other plants currently used in their herbal forms are as yet "undiscovered," or at least unavailable. Still, the herbs themselves are wonderful, and you can enjoy the fragrance of the oils as well as their healing properties in a simple cup of tea.

Components of Essential Oils

A plant contains a combination of natural chemical components, or constituents, that are responsible for its particular taste, smell and medicinal properties. Such components include alkaloids, saponins, tannins, glycosides, volatile oils, phytohormones, minerals and vitamins. The constituents that we are concerned with in aromatherapy are the volatile (essential) oils.

There are more than 30,000 known aromatic molecules. The number and combination of these molecules vary from plant to plant, making each essential oil unique. An essential oil usually contains about 100 different aromatic molecules, but the number may range between 10 and 500. Some have even more. This means that a given essential oil is not composed of just one type of molecule. Its composition is a complex array of components that gives each plant its characteristic odor and flavor, as well as accounting for its unique effects upon the consumer.

CHEMICAL GROUPS

Essential oils are mixtures of aromatic molecules built from three basic elements: carbon, hydrogen and oxygen. Depending on the type of molecules they contain, volatile oils are classified into different chemical or functional groups based on their constituents. These chemical groups characterize the nature of the whole molecule and its properties. The main groups are phenols, terpenes, alcohols, ketones, esters, ethers, oxides, aldehydes, coumarins and acids, although the acid group is not found in the essential oils. The actions of these chemical groups are explained below, along with examples of plants and the constituents of each group. Classifying essential oils according to the group of molecules most prevalent can be of great value in understanding the basic properties and actions of an oil, and allows us to understand how different oils can have the same basic properties and actions.

If you are unfamiliar with chemistry, envision an essential oil separated into segments, some larger and some smaller, each of which represents a different component. For instance, the essential oil of lemon thyme (a variety of thyme with a distinct lemon scent) smells like thyme because of the component thymol (found in many species of thyme), but also smells like lemon because it contains a component called citronellal.

Often the same aromatic molecule will be found in different plants. For example, rose, citronella, palmarosa and geranium all contain geraniol; cinnamon leaf and clove both contain eugenol. Similar essential oils can give unrelated plants very similar fragrances. Anise and star anise are a good example. Both smell and taste like licorice because both have the constituent anethole. Another example of unrelated plants with a similar fragrance is melissa and lemon verbena, both of which have citrus components (neral and geraniol) that give them a lemony smell. On the other hand, rosewood, coriander, French basil and lavender all contain linalol but smell very different due to the other constituents in their makeup.

Specific essential oils are often dominated by one or two types of molecules. Wintergreen, for example, can contain up to 99 percent methyl salicylate, mustard up to 95 percent allyl isothiocyanate; both are potentially hazardous. Sandalwood, a relatively safe oil, may contain 65 to 90 percent santalol. Clovebud oil may contain 70 to 80 percent eugenol. Exotic (Reunion) basil can contain up to 80 percent methyl chavicol, but the French (sweet) basil is high in linalol (40-45 percent) and has approximately 20 percent methyl chavicol. Both come from the same species, *Ocimum basilicum.*

Interestingly, the compound that predominates in an oil is not always the one responsible for most of its activity. The presence of trace components can significantly change the odor and flavor, and sometimes even the action, of an essential oil. Linalyl acetate and linalol make up about 90 percent of the aromatic molecules found in clary sage. A third molecule, sclareol, makes up only 5 to 7 percent, but is nonetheless responsible for the decidedly estrogenic action of the essential oil. Approximately 3 percent of clary sage oil is made up of some 300 other molecules. Mandarin is 95 percent terpenes; 74 other identified components make up the other 5 percent.

Many essential oils contain compounds from different aromatic families. Examples include helichrysum, which has esters and ketones; neroli, which has aldehydes and alcohols; and peppermint, which contains both alcohols and ketones. Rose is an example of a chemically complex plant, containing more than 400 different aromatic molecules, including esters, alcohols and acids. Rose geranium and lavender both have more than 350 molecules from a variety of biochemical groups, including alcohols, esters and aldehydes.

Plants extracted by the carbon-dioxide process are generally more complex than those derived by distillation, simply because that process extracts other components in addition to volatile oils.

The name of a chemical compound is often taken from the botanical or common name of a plant. Thymol comes from thyme, citronellal from citronella, pinene from pine, geraniol from geranium, bergaptene from bergamot. In some instances, the ending of a compound name can provide a hint as to what group it belongs in. For example, terpenes end in "ene," ketones end in "one," aldehydes end in "al," and both phenols and alcohols end in "ol."

Chemotypes

Chemotypes are a phenomenon of nature whereby plants from the same genus and species produce different aromatic molecules. The specific molecules produced by each plant are determined by genes and enzymes, both of which are influenced by weather and soil conditions, altitude and the subsequent variations in light wavelengths. Chemotypes are reproduced by cloning rather than pollination.

Thyme oil produced from *Thymus vulgaris* grown at sea level is high in thymol. The plant grown under these conditions produces different aromatic molecules than would a *Thymus vulgaris* plant grown in the mountains, which would be high in linalol. *Thymus vulgaris* has more than eight chemotypes. The different aromatic molecules in each chemotype define very specific applications for each oil, although they are all from the same species of plant. Chemotypes are specified thus: *Thymus vulgaris* linalol, *Thymus vulgaris* thymol, etc.

Most of the different eucalyptus oils (*Eucalyptus globulus, E. citriodora, E. radiata*) are not chemotypes, but are from different species. However, *Eucalyptus polybractea* does produce the chemotypes cryptone and cineol, each of which has different applications. *Eucalyptus dives* also produces two chemotypes, piperitone and cineol. *Rosmarinus officinalis* produces verbenone, "1,8" cineol and camphor.

Most of the chemical groups discussed below are made up of oxygenated compounds, which means that their molecules come with an oxygen atom attached. Terpenes, the exception, are hydrocarbon compounds, containing only hydrogen and carbon.

Phenols

This group contains the most stimulating, bactericidal and immune-modulating compounds of all the aromatic groups. Phenols are often irritating to the skin and toxic to the liver, and therefore should be used with caution, in low dilutions and only for short periods of time. Essential oils in the phenol group include clove, oregano, savory and specific chemotypes of thyme. Compounds include carvacrol, thymol, eugenol, gaiacol, chavicol and australol.

Terpenes

Terpenes are antiseptic and stimulating, but may be irritating to the skin in concentrated amounts. Essential oils that contain molecules from this group include lemon, orange, mastic, nutmeg, angelica, pine, black pepper and bergamot. Chemists differentiate subgroups of terpenes by the number of carbon atoms they contain. Monoterpene contain 10 carbon atoms, sesquiterpenes 15 carbon atoms. Diterpenes are C_{20} molecules, meaning they contain 20 carbon atoms. Some constituents in the monoterpene group include limonene, terpinene, camphene, myrcene, sabinene, p-cymene, phellandrene, a- and b-pinene, and thujene.

An important subgroup, the sesquiterpenes, are mainly distilled from roots and woods, or from plants of the Asteraceae family (formerly known as the Compositae family). Sesquiterpene compounds include caryophyllen (clove), whose actions are anti-inflammatory and antiviral; farnesol (rose and chamomile), which is antibacterial; chamazulene and bisabolol (tansy, yarrow, and chamomile), which are anti-inflammatory and analgesic; and valeranon (valerian), which is antispasmodic and sedative. Other sesquiterpenes include santalol (sandalwood), zingiberol (ginger), veriteron and vetiveral (vetiver), and carotol (carrot seed). Spikenard is almost 100 percent sesquiterpenes.

Diterpenes (20 carbon atoms) are rarely found in essential oils, and although terpenoid molecules with 30 to 40 carbon atoms do occur in plants (plant steroids and hormones), their molecular weight is too heavy to allow evaporation with steam.

Alcohols

Toning, stimulating, antibacterial and antiviral, alcohols are also energizing and generally nontoxic. Essential oils containing monoterpene alcohols include geranium, ravensare, rosewood, rose and tea tree. Completely nonirritating and safe to use, the beneficial constituents found in these plants include geraniol, menthol, a-terpineol, terpineol-4, sabinol, linalol (sometimes called linalool) and thuyanol. Monoterpenols include cinalol, geraniol, nerol, a-terpineol, cuminol, carveol, borneol, pinocarveol, sabinol and menthol. The object of much research and interest, sesquiterpenol molecules in the alcohol group are anti-inflammatory and stimulate immune responses. They include nerolidol (neroli), bisabolol (chamomile), carotol (carrot seed), a- and b-santalol (sandalwood), vetiverol (vetiver), sclareol (clary sage), zingiberol (ginger), patchoulol (patchouli) and farnesol (rose).

Ketones

The actions of ketones are mucolytic (dissolve mucus), cicatrizant (wound-healing) and lipolytic (dissolve fats). Potentially toxic ketones are found in sage, hyssop, pennyroyal and thuja. Their toxic effects vary depending on the plant, but oils in this group can have abortive, convulsive, stupefying or epileptic actions. Examples of fragrant molecules in the ketone group include thujone, carvone, menthone, atlantone, vetivone, pinocamphone, piperitone, cryptone, verbenone, jasmone, fenchone and pulegone. Subgroups include diones, such as those found in helichrysum, and cytotoxic lactones, which are contained in inula. Nontoxic oils in this group include jasmine, fennel, and, to some extent, peppermint.

Esters

A reaction product of acids and alcohols, esters are the most balancing of all the chemical families of essential oils. They are relaxing and soothing, and many have antispasmodic and antifungal properties. Oils that contain a good proportion of esters tend to smell very pleasant; these include lavender, bergamot, clary sage, ylang-ylang, Roman chamomile and marjoram. Examples of aromatic molecules in this group are linalyl acetate, neryl acetate, geranyl acetate, bornyl acetate and other acetates.

Plants in this category include basil, tarragon and cedar. The aromatic molecules are methyl chavicol, methyl eugenol, and cedryl methyl ether. These tend to have antispasmodic actions. Also included are the constituent transanethole, found in anise; apiol, found in parsley; and myristicin, found in nutmeg.

Oxides

Essential oils containing oxides include camphorous oils such as tea tree, naiouli, rosemary, cajeput, hyssop (variety decumbens), bay laurel and eucalyptus. The most important aromatic molecule in this group is "1,8" cineol, but it also includes piperitonoxide, bisabolol oxide, bisabolone oxide and linalol oxide. Within the oxide group there are potentially toxic molecules that can cause convulsions: asarone (from calamus) and ascaridol (found in wormseed oil). Menthofuran, which may be present in peppermint oil if the plant was harvested during flowering, is also toxic.

Aldehydes

Aldehydes are anti-inflammatory, calming, antiseptic and sedating, but also may be somewhat irritating to the skin if used undiluted. Many lemon-scented oils fall into this category, including lemongrass, melissa, lemon verbena, citronella and eucalyptus citriodora. Cinnamon bark is also in the aldehyde group, but has other irritating constituents. Examples of specific aromatic molecules include citral, geranial, neral, citronellal, myrtenal, phellandral, cinnamic aldehyde and benzaldehyde.

Coumarins

Coumarins have potentially toxic properties that can cause or contribute to liver damage or photosensitivity. They are also blood thinners. Therefore, they should be used with caution by people with problems in any of these areas, or for those who take blood-thinning medications. Examples of coumarins are bergaptene, herniarine, angelicine, citronene and furocoumarin. Oils in this group include bergamot, ammi visnaga, angelica, citruses and, to some extent, lavender.

Acids

Some essential oils contain acids, but the majority of acids (e.g., carboxylic, angelic and quinic acid) are found primarily in aromatic hydrosols. They are anti-inflammatory and antiseptic as well as moisturizing.

PART IV

Charts

Look in the perfumes of flowers and of nature for peace of mind and joy of life.

—Wang Wei

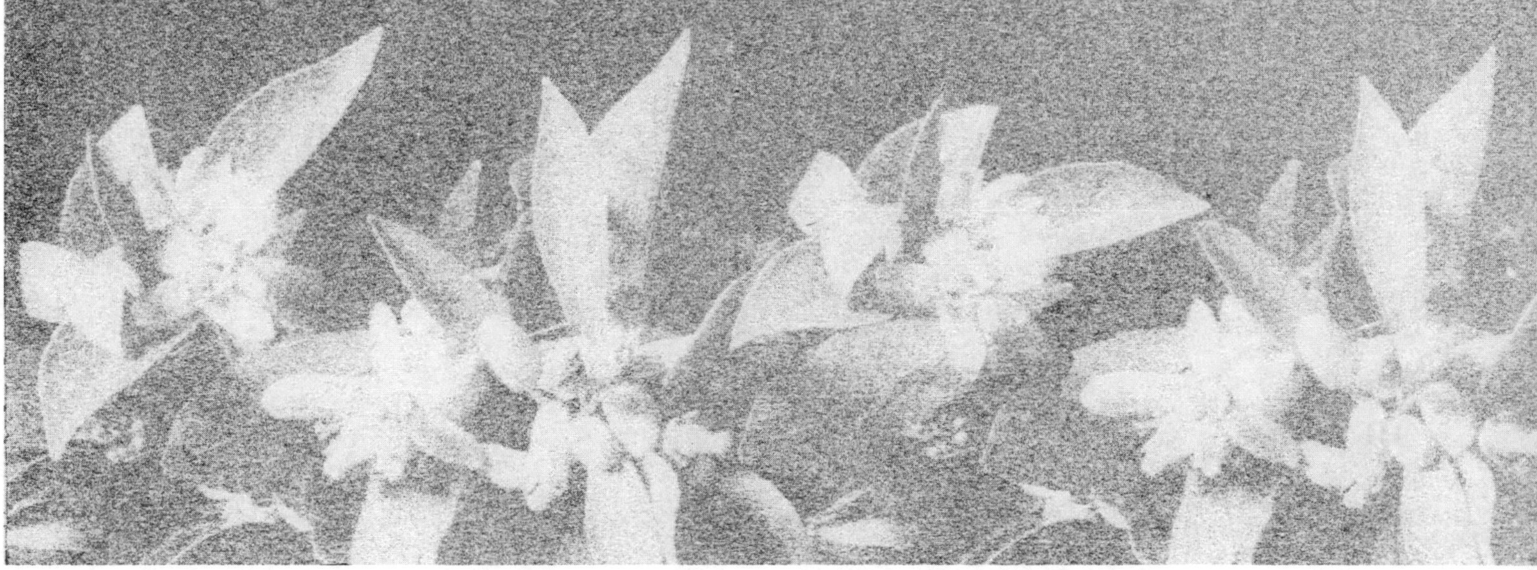

How to Use the Charts

The following charts distill the information presented in this book into an easy-to-use format. They will help you choose at a glance the best essential oils for your project. We think that the creative—and most fun—part of aromatherapy is designing your own formulas. These custom-made blends are also the most effective.

To use the charts, choose a condition you would like to treat and read down that column to see what oils are suggested. In most cases there are more oils listed than you need for one formula, so look up each one in Chapter 6: Materia Medica. Reading about all of the attributes of each oil will make it obvious which one is best suited for your blend. You can also base your selection on the availability of the oils, perhaps choosing ones that you already have, that are easily available or that fit your price range. Once your essential oil blend is completed information in Chapter 4: Guidelines for Using Essential Oils and Herbs will help you decide which base is the most appropriate to dilute the blend and the best way to use it.

You can also use these charts to learn more about a particular essential oil by reading across the column to see the conditions that it treats. This will help you choose which essential oils to purchase. You can also use these charts to help you put together an aromatherapy collection for a particular purpose, say for a first-aid kit or a complexion-care kit for a particular skin type. You may be surprised how many things you can do with just four or five different essential oils.

For the charts, we selected the essential oils that are used the most often. After you have some expertise in formulating, you will probably want to expand your selection to other essential oils and will may even find yourself making your own charts. We find that charts are not only an excellent learning tool, but are very handy even after you have been working with aromatherapy for years.

Fragrances for Emotions

(See Chapter 3: Scent and Psyche for more information.)

	ANGER	ANXIETY	APATHY	CONFUSION	DEPRESSION	FEAR	FORGETFULNESS	GRIEF	HYPER-SENSITIVE	IMPATIENCE	INSTABILITY	INSOMNIA	MELANCHOLY	PANIC/SHOCK	STRESS/OVERWORK	IRRITABILITY	KEY WORD
ANISE											X				X		THOUGHTFULL
BASIL	X	X		X	X	X	X								X		CONFIDENCE
BAY							X							X	X		PURPOSE
BENZOIN		X									X		X				PROTECTION
BERGAMOT		X			X					X	X	X			X		NON-COMPULSIVE
CAMPHOR		X		X						X	X			X			CENTERED
CARDAMOM		X		X											X		WARMTH
CEDAR				X					X							X	PURITY
CHAMOMILE	X	X			X	X			X	X	X	X		X	X		STAMINA
CLARY SAGE					X				X					X	X	X	EXHILARATION
CINNAMON	X			X												X	EVIGORATION
CORIANDER	X				X	X	X							X			PARANOIA
CYPRESS		X		X				X			X	X				X	PURPOSE
EUCALYPTUS									X					X	X		ENERGY
FENNEL		X				X				X					X		CLARITY
FRANKINCENSE	X	X		X	X					X		X	X		X		FAITH
GERANIUM	X	X	X		X				X		X	X					TRANQUILITY
HELICHRYSUM				X	X						X				X		FORTITUDE
HYSSOP	X			X		X		X	X		X						STRENGTH
JASMINE	X	X	X	X		X		X		X		X		X			FANTASY
JUNIPER		X							X						X		RENEWAL
LAVENDER	X	X		X	X				X	X	X	X	X	X	X		BALANCE
LEMON				X	X						X	X			X		CLEANLINESS
MARJORAM		X		X				X	X	X	X	X	X		X		COMFORT
MELISSA	X	X				X	X					X	X	X		X	STABILITY
MYRRH									X	X	X	X					DEVOTION
NEROLI	X		X	X	X	X			X			X			X	X	CONFIDENCE
NUTMEG		X										X			X		MINDLESS
ORANGE						X								X	X	X	HAPPINESS
PATCHOULY		X	X	X	X				X			X		X		X	COMPROMISE
PETITGRAIN		X			X							X		X			EXPANSION
PEPPERMINT		X	X	X	X								X	X	X		ENERGY
PINE	X	X	X		X												DIRECTION
ROSE	X	X	X		X	X		X	X	X		X	X		X		COMFORT
ROSEMARY		X	X				X	X			X		X				PERCEPTION
ROSEWOOD	X	X	X		X								X	X	X		CONSTRUCTIVE
SAGE			X					X				X			X		FOCUS
SANDALWOOD		X		X	X						X	X	X		X		INTENT
VETIVERT					X									X			GROUNDING
THYME						X					X		X		X		AWARENESS
YLANG-YLANG	X	X			X		X		X			X		X	X		ACCEPTANCE

Essential Oils for Physical Problems

(See Chapter 5: Therapeutics for more information.)

	CONSTIPATION	FEVER	GALL BLADDER	HEADACHES	HORMONAL	INDIGESTION	INFECTIONS	INSOMNIA	LUNG CONGESTION	MENSTRUATION	MUSCLE PAIN
ANISE			X		X	X					
BASIL		X			X	X	X		X	X	
BAY						X					X
BENZOIN							X		X		
BERGAMOT											
BLACK PEPPER	X	X				X	X				
CAMPHOR	X						X				X
CARROT											
CEDAR							X	X	X		
CHAMOMILE		X	X			X	X			X	X
CLARY SAGE											
CINNAMON	X					X	X				X
CYPRESS							X				
EUCALYPTUS		X	X		X		X		X	X	X
FENNEL	X				X	X	X			X	
FRANKINCENSE			X				X		X		
GERANIUM					X		X				
GINGER						X				X	X
HYSSOP		X					X		X		
JASMINE							X			X	
JUNIPER						X	X		X	X	X
LAVENDER			X			X	X	X			X
LEMON		X	X				X				
MARJORAM	X					X	X	X	X	X	X
MELLISA						X	X	X			
MYRRH						X	X		X	X	
NEROLI						X	X	X			
ORANGE						X	X				
PEPPERMINT	X	X				X	X		X	X	X
ROSE	X					X	X	X		X	
ROSEMARY	X					X	X			X	X
ROSEWOOD											
SAGE						X	X			X	
SANDALWOOD						X	X	X	X	X	
THYME						X	X		X	X	X
TEA TREE						X	X				

Essential Oils for Skin Problems

(See Chapter 5: Therapeutics for more information.)

	ALLERGIES	BITES	BOILS	BURNS	DERMATITIS	INFECTION—VIRAL	INFECTION—BACTERIAL	INFECTION—FUNGAL	INFLAMMATION	PAIN	REJUVENATION	RASHES/ITCHING	SCARS	SKIN GROWTHS	VEINS, ENLARGED	WARTS	WOUNDS
BASIL		X					X					X					
BENZOIN					X	X	X	X	X			X					X
BERGAMOT			X			X	X		X				X	X			X
CAMPHOR					X	X	X	X	X	X			X				
CEDAR		X			X		X					X					
CHAMOMILE	X	X	X	X	X	X	X		X	X	X	X	X	X	X		
CISTUS							X				X		X				X
CLARY SAGE											X						
CYPRESS	X				X							X		X			X
EUCALYPTUS		X	X			X	X	X		X		X					
FENNEL							X		X		X						
FRANKINCENSE			X				X	X	X				X	X			
GALBANUM					X	X		X									
GERANIUM		X		X			X	X	X	X	X	X			X		
HELICRHYSUM			X	X	X		X	X	X		X	X	X				X
JUNIPER		X			X		X		X			X		X	X		
LAVENDER	X	X		X	X	X	X	X	X	X	X	X	X	X	X	X	X
LEMON		X	X			X	X									X	X
LEMON GRASS							X		X								
MARJORAM		X		X		X	X	X	X	X	X						X
MELISSA	X	X			X	X	X										
MYRRH					X	X	X	X	X		X		X			X	X
NEROLI					X							X			X		
PATCHOULY							X	X	X	X	X	X					X
PEPPERMINT		X				X	X	X		X		X					
ROSE					X	X	X		X	X	X	X					
ROSEMARY		X			X	X	X	X	X	X	X		X		X		
ROSEWOOD				X						X			X				X
SAGE		X	X	X			X										
SANDALWOOD		X						X	X		X	X					
TEA TREE		X	X	X	X	X	X	X	X	X		X				X	
THUJA																X	
THYME		X			X		X	X								X	

Essential Oils for Hair Care

(See Chapter 8: Body Care for more information.)

	NORMAL HAIR	DRY HAIR	OILY HAIR	DANDRUFF	HAIR GROWTH	CLEANSING	HIGHLIGHTS	SCALP DERMATITIS
BASIL			X		X			
CEDAR			X		X			X
CHAMOMILE	X	X	X	X		X	X	X
CLARY SAGE		X	X	X		X		
CYPRESS			X					X
FENNEL			X			X		
GERANIUM	X	X	X	X		X		
JUNIPER			X	X			X	
LAVENDER	X	X	X	X		X		X
LEMON	X		X	X		X	X	
LEMON GRASS			X	X		X	X	
MYRRH		X		X				X
ORANGE			X					
PATCHOULY			X	X				
PEPPERMINT		X			X			
ROSE	X	X	X					
ROSEMARY	X	X	X	X	X			X
ROSEWOOD		X						
SAGE			X	X				
SANDALWOOD	X	X						X
SPIKENARD		X						
TEA TREE			X	X	X	X		X
THYME			X					X
YLANG-YLANG			X	X				

Essential Oils for Complexion Types

(See Chapter 9: Facial Care for more information.)

	NORMAL	DRY	OILY	COMBINATION	PROBLEM	COUPEROSE	MATURE	SUN-DAMAGED	SENSITIVE
BASIL			X						
BERGAMOT			X		X				
CARROT		X					X	X	
CEDAR			X		X				
CHAMOMILE	X	X		X	X	X		X	X
CISTUS		X			X		X		
CLARY SAGE		X	X		X		X		X
CYPRESS			X						
FENNEL		X	X				X		
FRANKINCENSE		X			X		X		X
EUCALYPTUS			X		X				
HELICRYSUM	X				X	X	X	X	X
GERANIUM	X	X	X	X	X	X	X		
JASMINE	X	X	X	X			X		X
JUNIPER			X		X				
LAVENDER	X	X	X	X	X	X	X	X	
LEMON			X		X				
LEMON GRASS			X		X				
MYRRH		X					X		X
NEROLI	X	X		X		X	X		X
ORANGE			X						
PALMA ROSA	X	X	X	X			X	X	
PATCHOULY			X		X		X		X
PEPPERMINT		X		X					
ROSE	X	X		X		X	X	X	X
ROSEMARY	X	X		X	X	X	X	X	
ROSEWOOD		X		X	X		X		X
SAGE			X		X				
SANDALWOOD	X	X	X	X	X				
SPIKENARD	X	X					X		
TEA TREE			X		X				
YLANG-YLANG			X	X	X				

Chemical Groups

(See Chapter 13: Chemistry for more information.)

Ketones *mucolytic, neurotoxic*	Thuja, Sage, Wormwood, Tansy, Hyssop, Camphor, Rosemary, Eucalyptus dives, Dill
Aldehydes *sedative*	Eucalyptus citriodora, Citronella, Lemon verbena, Melissa, Litsea cubeba, Cumin
Esters *balancing, soothing*	Lavender, Clary Sage, Roman Chamomile, Geranium, Ylang Ylang
Ethers *antispasmodic*	Basil, Tarragon, Anis Seed, Parsley, Nutmeg, Sassafras
Alcohols *tonifying, energizing*	Rosewood, Coriander, Petitgrain, Rose, Palmarosa, Eucalyp tus radiata, Neroli, Niaouli, Ravensare aromatica, Tea Tree, Marjoram, Peppermint, Spearmint
Phenols *stimulant, antibacterial*	Thyme, Oregano, Savory, Clove
Oxides *expectorant*	Eucalyptus globulus, Bay, Hyssop off. var. decumbens
Terpenes *drying, anti viral*	Orange, Lemon, Pine, Cypress, Spruce, Douglas Fir
Sesqui-terpenes *anti inflammative*	German Chamomile, Ginger, Sandalwood, Patchouli,

PART V

Appendices

Smell is a potent wizard that transports us across thousands of miles and all the years that we have lived.

—Helen Keller

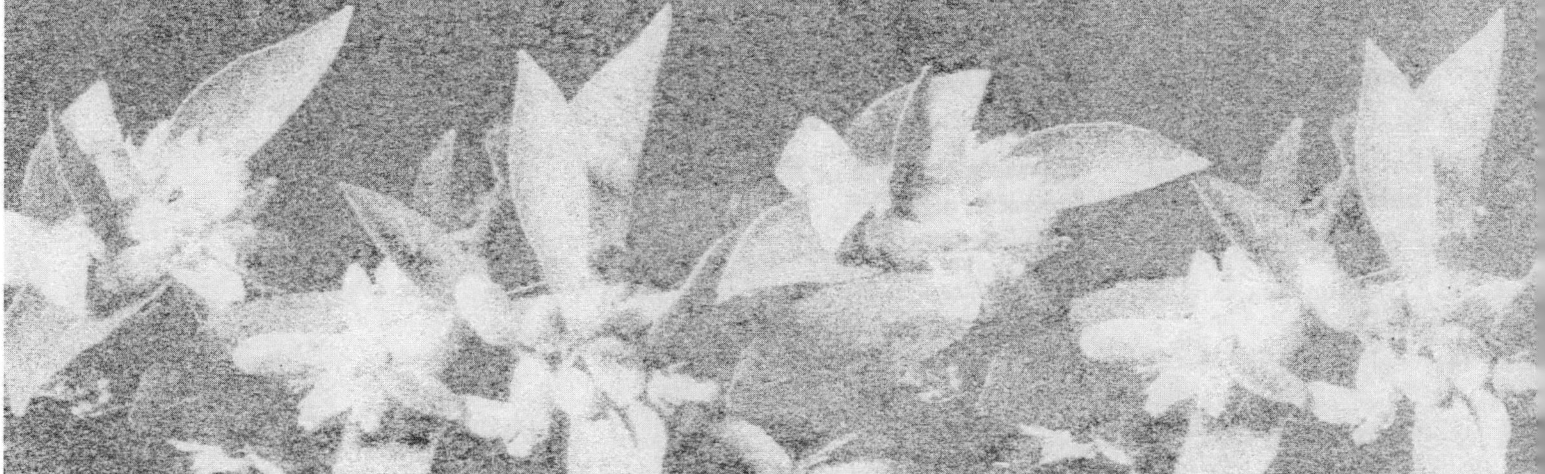

Botanical Names of Herbs

This cross reference gives the Latin herb names mentioned throughout the book. The Latin names of the essential oils are given in the Materia Medica.

A

Aloe Vera	*Aloe barbendensis*
Alkanet	*Alkanna tinctoria*
Astragalus	*Astragalus membranicus*
Arnica	*Arnica montana*

B

Barberry	*Berberis vulgaris*
Black Cohosh	*Cimicifuga racemosa*
Black Current	*Ribes nigrum*
Black Walnut	*Juglans nigra*
Blackberry	*Rubus* species
Bladderwrack	*Fucus vesiculosus*
Blue Cohosh	*Caulophyllum thalictroides*
Borage	*Borago offcinalis*
Burdock	*Arctium lappa*

C

Calendula	*Calendula officinalis*
California Poppy	*Escholzia californica*
Cascara	*Rhamnus purshianus*
Catnip	*Nepeta cataria*
Celery	*Apium graveolens*
Chaste Berry	*Vitex agnus-castus*
Chickweed	*Stellaria media*
Cleavers	*Galium aparine*
Comfrey	*Symphytum officinale*
Corn Silk	*Zea mays*
Cramp Bark	*Viburnum opulus*

D

Dandelion	*Taraxacum officinalis*
Devil's Claw	*Harpagophytum procumbens*
Dong Quai	*Angelica sinensis*

E

Echinacea	*Echinacea purpurea* or *E. angustifolia*
Elder	*Sambucus nigra*
Elecampane	*Inula helenium*

F

False Unicorn	*Chamaelirium luteum*
Fenugreek	*Trigonella foenum-graecum*
Flax Seed	*Linum usitatissimum*

G

Garlic	*Allium sativum*
Gentian	*Gentiana lutea*
Ginkgo	*Ginkgo biloba*
Ginseng	*Panax ginseng*
Golden Rod	*Solidago* species
Golden Seal	*Hydrastis canadensis*
Gotu Kola	*Centella asiatica*
Green Tea	*Thea sinensis*
Grindelia	*Grindelia* species

H

Hawthorn	*Crataegus laevigata*
Henna	*Lawsonia* species
Hops	*Humulus lupulus*
Horehound	*Marrubium vulgare*
Horsetail	*Equisetum arvense*
Horseradish	*Armoracia rusticana*

J

Jewelweed	*Impatiens capensis*

L

Lady's Mantle	*Alchemilla vulgaris*
Licorice	*Glycyrrhiza glabra*
Linden	*Tillia* species

M

Marshmallow	*Althea officinalis*
Meadowsweet	*Filipendula ulmaria*
Milk Thistle	*Silybum marianus*
Motherwort	*Leonurus cardiaca*
Mugwort	*Artemisia vulgaris*
Mullein	*Verbascum thapsus*
Mustard	*Brassica nigra*

N

Neem	*Azadirachta indica*
Nettle	*Urtica dioica*

O

Oregon Grape Root	*Mahonia aquifolium*

P

Parsley	*Pertoselinum crispum*
Partridge Berry	*Mitchella repens*
Passion Flower	*Passiflora incarnata*
Pau d'Arco	*Tabebuia* species
Plantain	*Plantago major* or *P. lanceolata*

R

Raspberry	*Rubus idaeus*
Red Clover	*Trifolium pratense*
Reishi Mushroom	*Ganoderma lucidum*

S

Safflower	*Carthamus tinctorius*
Sarsaparilla	*Smilax officinalis*
Sassafrass	*Sassafras albidum*
Saw Palmetto	*Serenoa serrulata*
Schizandra	*Schisandra chinensis*
Shepherds Purse	*Capsella bursa-pastoris*
Shiitake Mushroom	*Lentinula edodes*
Siberian Ginseng	*Eleutherococcus senticosus*
Slippery Elm	*Ulmus fulva*
Strawberry	*Fragaria vesca*
St. John's wort	*Hypericum perforatum*

U

Usnea	*Usnea barbata*
Uva Ursi	*Arctostaphylos uva ursi*

V

Valerian	*Valariana officinalis*
Vervain	*Verbena officinalis*

W

Willow	*Salix alba*
Wild Cherry Bark	*Prunus serotina*
Wild Indigo	*Baptisia tinctoria*
Wild Lettuce	*Lactuca virosa*
Wild Oat	*Avena sativa*
Wild Yam	*Dioscorea villosa*
Witch Hazel	*Hamamelis virginiana*

Y

Yarrow	*Achillea millifolium*
Yellow Dock	*Rumex crispus*

Aromatherapy Resources

Associations and Journals

American Herb Association
P.O. Box 1673
Nevada City, CA 95959
Newsletter: *AHA Quarterly*
Includes articles on aromatherapy.

Canadian Federation of Aromatherapists
Box 68571-1235 Williams Parkway-East
Brampton, Ontario Canada L6S 6A1
Newsletter: *Escential News*

American Herbalist Guild
P.O. Box 1683
Soquel, CA 95073
Newsletter: *The Herbalist*

The International Federation of Aromatherapists
46 Dalkeith Rd.
London, England SE21, 8LS

International Journal of Aromatherapy and
American Alliance of Aromatherapy
P.O. Box 750428
Petaluma, CA 94975-0428
(707) 769-5120
Newsletter: *News Quarterly*

National Association for Holistic Aromatherapy
219 Carl St.
San Francisco, CA 94117
Newsletter: *Scentsitivity*

The Association of Tisserand Aromatherapists
65 Church Rd.
Hove, East Sussex England BN3 2BD

Education Aromatherapy

Carol Corio
9 Demars
Maynard, MA 01754
(800) 688-8343

Dorene Petersen
Aromatherapy Cetificate Home Study
Australasian College of Herbal Studies
P.O. Box 57
Lake Oswego, OR 97034
(800) 648-STUDY
Correspondence course

Jeanne Rose
Aromatherapy Study Course
219 Carl St.
San Francisco, CA 94117
Correspondence course and seminars
Catalog: $2

Kurt Schnaubelt
The Aromatherapy Course
P.O. Box 6723
San Rafael, CA 94903
Correspondence courses and seminars

Michael Scholes
Aromatherapy Seminars
3370 South Robertson Blvd.
Los Angeles, CA 90034
(800) 677-2368
Correspondence course and seminars
Newsletter: *Beyond Scents*

Mindy Green
c/o Rocky Mt. Center for Botanical Studies
P.O. Box 19254
Boulder, CO 80308-2254
Herb and aromatherapy seminars, private consulting, product development

Kathi Keville
Oak Valley Herb Farm
P.O. Box 2482
Nevada City, CA 95959
Herb and aromatherapy seminars

Galina Lisin
True Science of Aromatherapy
25063 Oak Ridge Ct.
Hayward, CA 94541
(510) 886-7729

Victoria Edwards
Leydet Aromatics
P.O. Box 2354
Fair Oaks, CA 95628
(916) 965-7546

John Steele
3949 Longridge Ave.
Sherman Oaks, CA 91423
(918) 789-2610

Herbal Correspondence Courses

Rosemary Gladstar
The Science and Art of Herbalism
P.O. Box 420
East Barre, VT 05649

David Hoffmann
Therapeutic Herbalism
2068 Ludwig Rd.
Santa Rosa, CA 95407

Essential Oil Suppliers

Aroma Land
Rt. 20, Box 29AL
Santa Fe, NM 87505
(800) 933-5267
Aroma jewelry and lamps

Herba Aromatica
25063 Oak Ridge Ct.
Hayward, CA 94541
(510) 886-7729
Aromatogram, essential oils, hydrosols

Oak Valley Herb Farm
P.O. Box 2482
Nevada City, CA 95959
Essential oils, aromatherapy massage bath and body oils, cosmetics, herbal products
Catalog $1

Original Swiss Aromatics
P.O. Box 6723
San Rafael, CA 94903
Essential oils, base ingredients, cosmetics, natural soap and shampoo base

Prima Fleur Botanicals
1201-R Anderson Dr.
San Rafael, CA 94901
(415) 455-0956
Essential Oils

Simpler Botanical Co.
P.O. Box 39
Forestville, CA 95436
Hydrosols, essential oils, carrier oils, herbal extracts and cosmetics

Victoria Edwards
Leydet Aromatics
P.O. Box 2354
Fair Oaks, CA 95628
(916) 965-7546

For a complete and current listing of courses and products:

The AHA Directory of Mail Order Herbal & Aromatherapy Products. $4.

The AHA Directory of Herbal Education (Includes aromatherapy). $3.50.

The AHA List of Recommended Books. $2.

The American Herb Association
P.O. Box 1673
Nevada City, CA 95959

Recommended Cosmetics Companies

Most of these can be found at natural food stores:

Alexandra Avery
Aroma Avery
Aubrey Organics
Botanics of California
Dr. Hauschka
Herba Aromatica
Geremy Rose
Paul Penders
Santa Fe Fragrance Co.
Weleda
Zia Cosmetics

Essential Oils Stills

Pope Scientific, Inc.
P.O. Box 495
Menomenee Falls, WI 53052-0495
(414) 251-9300

Essential Oil Quality Analysis

Spectrix
Division of Body Love, Inc.
303 Potrero #31
Santa Cruz, CA 95060
(408) 425-8218

Essential Oil Professional Resources

The Journal of Essential Oil Research
Allured Publishing Corporation
362 S. Schmale Rd.
Carol Stream, IL 60188
(708) 653-2155

Perfumer and Flavorist (Journal)
Allured Publishing Corporation
2100 Manchester Rd., Bldg. C, Suite 1600
Wheaton, IL 60187

U.S. Essential Oil Trade
1993 Publication, Circular Series
U.S. Department of Agriculture
Foreign Agricultural Service
Room 4655-S
Washington, DC 20250-1000

The Flavor and Extract Manufacturers' Association
of the United States
FEMA
900 17th St., NW
Washington, DC 20006

Bibliography

Al-Samarqandi. *The Medical Formulary*. (13th century) Reprint. Levey, Martin and Noury, LaKhaledy, Eds. Oxford University Press, 1967.

Alpers, William C. *The Era Formulary*. D.O. Hayes & Co., 1914.

Arctander, Steffen. *Perfume and Flavor Materials of Natural Origins*. Self-published, 1960.

Atal and Kapur, ed. *Cultivation and Utilization of Aromatic Plants*. India: Regional Research Lab., Council of Scientific & Industrial Research, India, 1982.

Bauer, Garbe and Surburg. *Common Fragrance and Flavor Materials*. Germany: VCH, 1990.

Carper, Jean. *The Food Pharmacy*. Bantam Books, 1988.

Chase, Deborah. *The Medically Based No-Nonsense Beauty Book*. Alfred A. Knopf, 1975.

Cooke, Kramer and Rowland-Entwistle. *History's Timeline*. Crescent Books, 1981.

Cooley, Arnold J. *The Toilet and Cosmetic Arts in Ancient and Modern Times*. Burt Franklin, 1970. (Originally publ. 1866.)

Craker, Lyle. E. & James E. Simon, Eds. *Herbs, Spices and Medicinal Plants: Recent Advances in Botany, Horticulture, and Pharmacy*. Vol. 1. Oryx Press., 1986.

D'Andrea, Jeanne. *Ancient Herbs*. California: J. Paul Getty Museum, 1982.

Donato, Giuseppe and Seefried, Monique. *The Fragrant Past: Perfumes of Cleopatra and Julius Caesar*. Italy: Instituto Poligrafico E Zecca Dello Stato, 1989.

Dorland, Wayne E. *The Flavors and Fragrance Industry*. Eng.: WED Co., 1977.

Duraffourd, Paul. *The Best of Health Thanks to Essential Oils*. La Vie Claire, 1984.

Engen, Trygg. *The Perception of Odors*. Academic Press, 1982.

Fischer-Rizzi, Susanne. *The Complete Aromatherapy Handbook*. Sterling, 1991.

Gattefosse, Rene-Maurice. *Gattefosse's Aromatherapy*. Eng: C.W. Daniel, 1993.

Genders, Roy. *Perfume Through the Ages*. Putnam, 1972.

Gerard, John. *The Herball or Generall Historie of Plants*. (1597). Enlarged by Thomas Johnson, 1636.

Gibbons, Boyd. The Intimate Sense. *National Geographic*. Sept. 1986.

Gilbert, Avery N. and Charles J. Wysocki. "The Smell Survey Results." *National Geographic*, 1987.

Gloss *et al.* Johnson Pub. Ltd., 1984.
The H & R Book of Perfume.
Fragrance Guide Feminine Notes.
Fragrance Guide Masculine Notes.
Guide to Fragrance Ingredients.

Guenther, Ernest. *The Essential Oils. Vols. I-IV*. Robert E. Kriefer Pub., 1948 (reprinted 1972).

Greer, Mary. *The Essence of Magic: Tarot, Ritual, and Aromatherapy*. Newcastle Pub., 1993.

Grieve, Maude. *A Modern Herbal, Vols. I-II*. Dover, 1971.

Gumbel, Dietrich. *Principles of Holistic Skin Therapy with Herbal Essences*. Jarl F. Haug Pubs., 1986.

Hildegard. *Manuscript*. (12th century) Reprint. Strenlow, Wighard and Gottfried, Herzka, Eds. Bear & Co., 1987.

Howes, David. "New Guinea: An Olfactory Ethnography" In *Dragoco Report*, 2, 1992:71-81.

Kaufman, William. *Perfume*. New York: E.P. Dutton, 1974.

Keville, Kathi, Ed. *The American Herb Association Quarterly*. Vols. 7:1-10:1. American Herb Association, 1988-1994.

Keville, Kathi. *Herbs: An Illustrated Encyclopedia*. Friedman/Fairfax,1992.

Landing, James E. *American Essence: History of the Peppermint & Spearmint Industry in the U.S.* Kalamazoo Public Museum, 1969.

Lautie, Raymond and Andre Passebecq. *Aromatherapy: The Use of Plant Essences in Healing*. Eng: Thorsans, 1979.

Lavabre, Marcel. *Aromatherapy Workbook*. New York: Inner Traditions, 1989.

Lawless, Julia. *The Encyclopedia of Essential Oils*. Massachusetts: Element Books, 1992.

LeGuerer, Annick. *Scent: The Mysterious and Essential Powers of Smell*. Turtle Bay Books, 1992.

Leuang, Albert Y. *Encyclopedia of Common Natural Ingredients Used in Food, Drugs and Cosmetics*. Wiley-Interscience, 1983.

Maury, Marguerite. *Marguerite Maury's Guide to Aromatherapy: The Secret of Life & Youth*. London: C. W. Daniel, 1989.

Morris, Edwin T. *Fragrance: The Story of Perfume from Cleopatra to Chanel*. Charles Scribner's, 1984.

Parry, Ernest.
The Chemistry of Essential Oils and Artificial Perfumes. Vols. I-II. Eng: Scott, Greenwood and Son, 1918.
Parry's Cyclopedia of Perfumery. Vols. I-II. Eng: Blakiston, 1925.

Piesse, G.W. Septimus. *The Art of Perfumery: Odors of Plants*. Presley Blakiston, 1880.

Poucher, William. *Perfumes, Cosmetics and Soaps*. Van Nostrand, 1926.

Pool, Lawrence J. *Nature's Masterpiece:The Brain and How It Works*. Walker and Co., 1987.

Rose, Jeanne. *The Aromatherapy Book*. North Atlantic Books, 1992.

Sacks, Dr. Oliver. *The Man Who Mistook His Wife for a Hat*. Eng: Duckworth Simmel, Georg, 1985.

Schnaubelt, Kurt. *The Aromatherapy Course*. San Rafael, California: Self-published, 1985.

School of Salernum. *Regimen Sanitatis Salernitanum*. (Illuminated 14th-century text). Reprint. JB Lippincott and Co., Trans., 1870.

Teranishi, Roy, Ron G. Buttery, & Hiroshi Sugisawa, Eds. *Bioactive Volatile Compounds from Plants*. American Chemical Society, 1993.

Theophrastus. *Enquiry Into Plants. 2 Vols*. (Concerning Odors) Reprint. Sir Arthur Hort, Trans., 1916. (Originally published 4th century BC.)

Tisserand, Robert.
Aromatherapy: To Heal and Tend the Body. Lotus Press, 1988.
The Essential Oil Safety Data Manual. England. Self-published, 1985.

Toller & Dodd, ed. *Perfumery. The Psychology and Biology of Fragrance*. Chapman & Hall, 1988.

Valnet, Jean. *The Practice of Aromatherapy*. Inner Traditions, 1980.

Verey, Rosemary. *The Scented Garden: Choosing and Using the Plants that Bring Fragrance to Your Life, Home and Table*. Van Nostrand.

Vogel, Vergil J. *American Indian Medicine*. University of Oklahoma Press, 1970.

Whitfield, Dr. Philip and D.M. Stoddart. *Hearing, Taste and Smell. Pathways to Perception*. Torstar Books, 1984.

Windhoiz, Martha, *et al.* Eds. *The Merck Index. An Encyclopedia of Chemicals and Drugs*. Merck & Co. 16th ed., 1992.

Winter, Ruth.
The Smell Book: Scents, Sex, and Society. J.B. Lippincott Co. 1976.
A Consumer's Dictionary of Cosmetic Ingredients. Crown Pub. (3rd edition), 1989.

Woolley, S.W. and Forrester. *Pharmaceutical Formulas. 2 Vols*. Eng: The Chemist and Druggist, 1929.

Worwood, Valerie. *The Complete Book of Essential Oils and Aromatherapy*. Eng: New World Library, 1990.

Wren, R.C. *Potter's New Cyclopedia of Botanical Drugs and Preparations*. Eng: The C.W. Daniel Co., 1985.

Scientific Resources

If you are interested in pursuing more scientific information on essential oils and aromatherapy, these studies can be obtained through a university library or through computer searches.

The Sense of Smell: Physical Properties of Essential Oils

A Behavioral Augmentation of Natural Immunity: Odor Supports a Pavlovian Conditioning Model, by H.B. Solvason, *et al.*, *International Journal of Neuroscience.*

The Intimate Sense of Smell, by B. Gibbons, *National Geographic,* Sept., pp. 324-360. 1986.

Magnitude and Category Scales of the Pleasantness of Odors, by T. Eugene and D. McBurney. *Journal of Experimental Psychology,* Vol. 68, pp. 435-40. 1964.

Marketing Scents . . . , by T. Green, *Smithsonian,* June, pp. 53-61. 1991.

Menstrual Synchrony and Suppression, by M.N. McClintock, *Nature,* Vol. 299, pp. 244-5. 1971.

New Guinea: An Olfactory Ethnography, by D. Howes, *Dragoco Report,* Vol. 2, pp. 71-81. 1992.

Odors and Private Language: Observations on the Phenomenology of Scent, by U. Almagor, *Human Studies,* Vol. 13, pp. 106-21. 1990.

Olfaction and the Right Cerebral Hemisphere, by D. Hines, *Journal of Altered States of Consciousness,* Vol. 3(1), pp. 47-59. 1977.

The Sense of Smell Awakens Nostalgia, by J. Jesse, *Dragoco Report,* Vol. 3, p. 76. 1982.

Sentimental Journeys, by P. Weintraub, *Omni,* Vol. 8(7), pp. 48-52. 1986.

A Sequential Contract Effect in Odor Perception, by H.T. Lawless, *Bulletin of the Psychonomic Society,* Vol. 29(4), pp. 317-19. 1991.

A Sociology of Smell, by A. Synnot, *Canadian Review of Sociology and Anthropology,* Vol. 28(4), pp. 437-459. 1991.

Taste and Smell: The Neglected Senses, by T. Ziporyn, *Journal of the American Medical Association,* Vol. 247(3), pp. 277-85. 1982.

This and That: The Essential Pharmacology of Herbs and Spices, by B. Max, *Trends in Pharmacological Sciences,* Vol. 13, pp. 15-20. 1992.

Unconscious Odor Conditioning in Human Subjects, by M.D. Kirk-Smith, C. Van Toller and G.H. Dodd, *Biological Psychology,* Vol. 100, pp. 221-3. 1983.

Scent and the Psyche: Emotional Properties of Essential Oils

Aromatherapy and Aerosols, by P.P. Rovesti, *Soap, Perfumery, and Cosmetics, Vol.* 46, pp. 47-57. 1973.

Aromatherapy and Occupational Therapy, by H. Sanderson and J. Ruddle, *British Journal of Occupational Therapy,* Vol. 55(8), pp. 310-314.

Aromatherapy: Evidence for Sedative Effects of the Essential Oil of Lavender After Inhalation, by G. Buchbauer, *et al., Journal of Biosciences,* Vol. 46(11-120), pp. 1067-72. 1991.

The Biology and Psychology of Perfume, by G.H. Dodd and C. Von Toller. *Perfumer and Flavorist,* 8, Vols. 1-14. 1983.

Central Neurotropic Effects of Lavender Essence, by S. Atanassova-Shopova and K. Roussinov. *Izv. Inst. Fiziol. Bulg. Akademia Nauk.,* Vol. 13, pp. 69-77. 1970.

CNV Brain Wave Patterns, By T.A. Lorig and M. Roberts, *Chemical Senses,* Vol. 15(5) pp. 537-545. 1990.

Complementary Therapy in Practice, by D. Crowther, *Nursing Standard,* Vol. 5(23), pp. 25-7. 1991.

The Effect of Olfactory Stimulation on Fluency, Vividness of Imagery and Associated Mood, by A. Roberts and J.M. Williams, *British Journal of Medical Psychology,* Vol. 65(2), pp. 197-199. 1992.

Effects of Olfactory Stimulation on Performance and Stress in a Visual Sustained Attention Task, by J.S. Warm, *et al., Journal of the Society of Cosmetic Chemists,* Vol. 42, pp. 199-210. 1991.

Effects . . . on Long-Term Memory for Odours, by M. Lyman and M.A. McDaniel. *Quarterly of the Journal of Experimental Psychology,* Vol. 38, pp. 753-65. 1986.

Effects of *Salvia Sclarea* Essential Oil on the Central Nervous System, by S. Atanassova-Shopova and K. Roussinov. *Izv. Inst. Fiziol. Bulg. Akademia Nauk.* Vol. 13, pp. 89-95. 1970.

Fragrance Compounds and Essential Oils with Sedative Effects Upon Inhalation, by G. Buchbauer, *et al., Journal of Pharmaceutical Sciences,* Vol. 82(6), pp. 660-664. 1993.

Experimental Inquiry into the Sedative Properties of Some Aromatic Drugs and Fumes, by D. Macht and Giu Ching Ting. *Journal of Experimental Therapeutics,* Vol. 18(5), pp. 361-72. 1921.

Have Scents to Relax?, by J.R. King, *World Medicine,* Vol. 19, pp. 29-31. 1983.

Longterm Memory of Odours . . . , by T. Engen, *et al., Journal of Experimental Psychology,* Vol. 100, p. 288. 1973.

Notes on the Unconscious Significance of Perfume, by J. Pratt, *International Journal of Psychoanalysis,* Vol. 23, pp. 80-3. 1942.

Neurophysical Effect of Bulgarian Essential Oils from Rose, Lavender and Geranium, by T. Tasev, *et al., Folia Medica,* Vol. 11 (5), pp. 307-17. 1969.

Observations of Eldercare in the USSR, by L. Duncan, *Geriatric Nursing,* Vols. 7-8. pp. 257-259. 1982.

Psychic Reactions to Olfactory Stimuli, by C.D. Daly and R.S. White. *British Journal of Medical Psychology*, Vol. 10, pp. 70-87. 1930.

Physiological/Psychological Background to the Reaction to Fragrance, by U. Harder, *Contact*, Vol. 32, pp. 14-22. 1984.

Sentimental Journey, Stress Management in Dermatology Patients, M. Marshall, *Nursing Standards*, Vol. 5(24), pp. 29-31. 1991.

Body: The Physical Properties of Essential Oils

Aromatherapy: Do Essential Oils Have Therapeutic Properties?, by G. Buchbauer, *Perfumer and Flavorist*, Vol. 15, pp. 47-50. 1990.

The Anti-Motion Sickness Mechanism of Ginger, by S. Holtmann et al., *Acta Oto-Laryngologica*, Vol. 108(3-4), pp. 168-74. 1989.

Antimicrobial Activity of Chamomile Oil, by M.E. Aggag and R.T. Yousef, *Planta Medica*, Vol. 22. pp. 140-44.

The Antiseptic Properties of Tea Tree Oil on Acne, by Bassett, I.B., *et al. The Medical Journal of Australia*, Vol. 153, pp. 455-58. 1990.

Antibacterial Evaluation of . . . Medicinal Volatile Oils, by A. Kar and S.R. Jain, *Qual. Plant Materia Vegetable*, Vol. 20(3), pp. 231-7. 1971.

Aroma Preservative: Essential Oils and Fragrances as Anti-Microbial Agents, by J. Kabara, *Cosmetic Sciences*, Vol. 1, pp. 237-73. 1984.

Caraway Oil Inhibits Skin Tumors, by M.H. Shwaireb, *Nutrition and Cancer*, Vol. 19(3), pp. 321-25. 1992.

Carminative Actions of Volatile Oils, by N. Harries, *et al.*, *Journal of Clinical Pharmacy*, Vol. 2, pp. 171-77. 1978.

Effect of Lemongrass on . . . *E. Coli Cells*, by E.O. Oguniana, *et al.*, *Microbios*, Vol. 50(202), pp. 43-59.

Effect of Peppermint and Eucalyptus Oil on . . . Headache, by H. Gobel, *et al.*, *Cephalalgia*, Vol 14(3), pp. 228-34. 1994.

Fungitoxicity of Essential Oils Against Dermatophytes, by N. Kishore, *et al.*, *Mycoses*, Vol. 36(5-6), pp. 211-5. 1993.

Germicidal Properties of the Essential Oil of *Melaleuca alternifolia* . . . , by P. Belaiche, *Phytothérapie*, Vol. 15, pp. 9-11. 1985.

The *in vitro* Antibacterial Activity of Essential Oils . . . , by J.C. Maruzella and P.A. Henry, *Journal of the American Pharmaceutical Association*, Vol. 47, pp. 294-6. 1958.

In vitro Antifungal Activity of Essential Oils . . . , by E.O. Lima, *et al.*, *Mycoses*, Vol. 36(9-10), pp. 333-36. 1993.

In vitro . . . Photosensitizing Properties of Bergamot Oil, by P. Morliere, *Journal of Photochemistry and Photobiology*, Vol. 7(2-4), pp. 199-208. 1990.

Study of the Antimicrobial Action of Various Essential Oils . . . , by P.J. Raharivelomana, *et al.*, *Archives de l'Institut Pasteur de Madagascar*, Vol. 56(1), pp. 261-71. 1989.

Treating Irritable Bowel Syndrome with Peppermint Oil, by W.D.W., *et al.*, *British Medical Journal*, Vol. 2, p. 835. 1979.

Treatment of Influenza with Volatile Oils Extracted from Chinese Plants, by S.G. Ong, *Science Record*, Vol. 2(7), pp. 233-8. 1958, and Vol. 3(3), pp. 120-7. 1959.

UV Sunscreen Properties in *Helichrysum*, by G. Prospero, Cosmet. and Toil., Vol. 91(3), p. 42. 1976.

Recommended Reading—Herb Books

Eastern/Central Medicinal Plants, by Steven Foster and James A. Duke. Houghton Mifflin Co., 1990.

Foundations of Health: The Liver & Digestive Herbal, by Christopher Hobbs. Botanica Press, 1992.

Herbal Healing for Women, by Rosemary Gladstar. Simon & Schuster, 1993.

Herbs and Health, by Kathi Keville. Rodale Press, 1996.

Herbs: An Illustrated Encyclopedia, by Kathi Keville. Friedman/Fairfax, 1992.

Herbs: American Country Living, by Kathi Keville. Crescent Books (Random House), 1991.

Herbs for Life, by Leslie Tierra. The Crossing Press, 1992.

Hygeia, by Jeannine Parvati. Freestone, 1978.

The Male Herbal, by James Green. The Crossing Press, 1991.

Medicinal Plants of the Pacific West, by Michael Moore. Red Crane Books, 1993.

The New Age Herbalist, by Richard Mabey. Collier Books/Macmillan Pub. Co., 1988.

The New Holistic Herbal, by David Hoffmann.

The New Healing Yourself: Natural Remedies for Adults and Children, by Joy Gardner. The Crossing Press, 1989.

Planetary Herbology, by Michael Tierra. Lotus Press, 1988.

Smart Medicine for a Healthier Child, by Janet Zand, Rachel Walton and Bob Rountree. 1994.

Wise Women Herbal for the Childbearing Years, by Susun Weed. Ash Tree Publishing, 1985.

Index

F

G

H

I

J

About the Authors

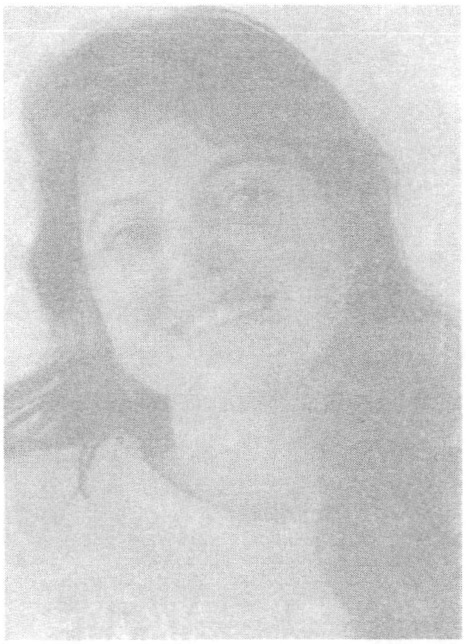

Kathi Keville has studied herbs since 1969. Her attraction to fragrant plants led to an involvement in aromatherapy. Her other books include *Herbs for Health and Healing; The Illustrated Encyclopedia of Herbs*; and *Herbs: American Country Living*. Keville is editor of the *American Herb Association Quarterly*, an honorary life member of the American Aromatherapy Association, a member of the National Institute of Holistic Aromatherapy, and a founding professional member of the American Herbalist Guild. She also is a masseuse and owns a mail-order herb business specializing in aromatherapy cosmetics. She travels throughout North America teaching seminars.

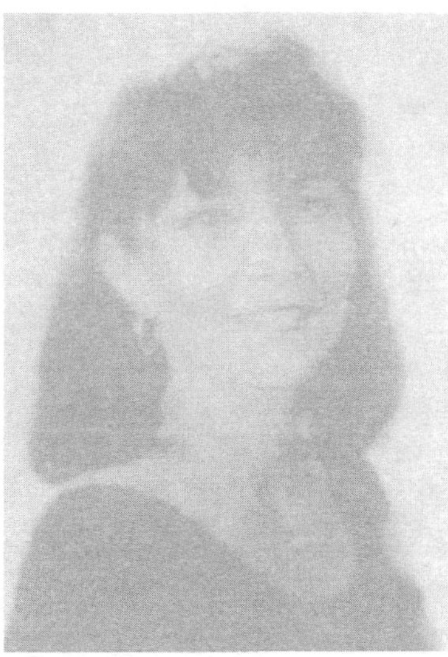

Mindy Green is an herbalist, massage practitioner, and esthetician. With twenty-three years' experience studying plants and their healing powers, Green now specializes in the study of aromatherapy and is a consultant in the industry. She is co-founder of Simpler's Botanical Co., a founding member of the American Herbalist Guild, and associate editor of the *American Herb Association Newsletter*. As co-director and faculty member of the California School of Herbal Studies and the Rocky Mountain Center for Botanical Studies, Green has lectured across the United States and Canada.